DENTOGIST

IVth Year BDS Question Bank (NTRUHS–Andhra Pradesh)

- Oral Medicine
- Oral and Maxillofacial Surgery
- Periodontics
- Endodontics
- Orthodontics
- Removable Partial Dentures
- Oral Radiology
- Local Anesthesia
- Operative Dentistry
- Pedodontics
- Complete Dentures
- Fixed Partial Dentures

Gopala Krishna BR BDS (MDS Ortho)
Davangere, Karnataka
India

Co-Author
Neha Chaphekar BDS
Bengaluru, Karnataka
India

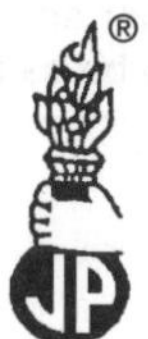

JAYPEE BROTHERS MEDICAL PUBLISHERS (P) LTD

Bengaluru • St Louis (USA) • Panama City (Panama) • New Delhi • Ahmedabad
Chennai • Hyderabad • Kochi • Kolkata • Lucknow • Mumbai • Nagpur

Published by
Jitendar P Vij
Jaypee Brothers Medical Publishers (P) Ltd

Corporate Office
4838/24 Ansari Road, Daryaganj, **New Delhi** - 110002, India, Phone: +91-11-43574357, Fax: +91-11-43574314

Registered Office
B-3 EMCA House, 23/23B Ansari Road, Daryaganj, **New Delhi** - 110 002, India
Phones: +91-11-23272143, +91-11-23272703, +91-11-23282021
+91-11-23245672, Rel: +91-11-32558559, Fax: +91-11-23276490, +91-11-23245683
e-mail: jaypee@jaypeebrothers.com, Website: www.jaypeebrothers.com

Offices in India

- **Ahmedabad**, Phone: Rel: +91-79-32988717, e-mail: ahmedabad@jaypeebrothers.com
- **Bengaluru**, Phone: Rel: +91-80-32714073, e-mail: bangalore@jaypeebrothers.com
- **Chennai**, Phone: Rel: +91-44-32972089, e-mail: chennai@jaypeebrothers.com
- **Hyderabad**, Phone: Rel:+91-40-32940929, e-mail: hyderabad@jaypeebrothers.com
- **Kochi**, Phone: +91-484-2395740, e-mail: kochi@jaypeebrothers.com
- **Kolkata**, Phone: +91-33-22276415, e-mail: kolkata@jaypeebrothers.com
- **Lucknow**, Phone: +91-522-3040554, e-mail: lucknow@jaypeebrothers.com
- **Mumbai**, Phone: Rel: +91-22-32926896, e-mail: mumbai@jaypeebrothers.com
- **Nagpur**, Phone: Rel: +91-712-3245220, e-mail: nagpur@jaypeebrothers.com

Overseas Offices

- **North America Office, USA,** Ph: 001-636-6279734, e-mail: jaypee@jaypeebrothers.com, anjulav@jaypeebrothers.com
- **Central America Office, Panama City, Panama,** Ph: 001-507-317-0160, e-mail: cservice@jphmedical.com Website: www.jphmedical.com

Dentogist: IVth Year BDS Question Bank (NTRUHS–Andhra Pradesh)

First Edition: **2010**

ISBN 978-81-8448-845-6

Typeset at JPBMP typesetting unit

Printed at Rajkamal Electric Press, Plot No. 2, Phase-IV, Kundli, Haryana.

DENTOGIST

IVth Year BDS Question Bank
(NTRUHS–Andhra Pradesh)

To

All the PG Students of Orthodontics
College of Dental Sciences (CODS)
Davangere, Karnataka, India

Preface

Every student's motive in life is to excel in the examinations with flying colours. But this is not as easy task without a proper guidance.

In order to show your complete caliber in examinations you need to have a planned systematic approach. 'You should not work hard but always should work smart'.

Usually in examinations 90% questions will be repetitive and if you cover up those questions, definitely you can hit the target easily.

This question bank includes all the questions appeared in the previous examinations with standard reference books along with page numbers which will make the work easy for students.

Only a student can understand other student needs and requirements, so this book is a complete package of those needs and demands. I hope this book can fulfill all the requirements of a student for the easy exam preparation.

Wishing you all the best.

Gopal Krishna BR

Contents

ORAL MEDICINE

SYLLABUS

1. Scope and importance of the subject
2. Methods of diagnosis including special investigations
3. Acute infections of the oral and paraoral structures
4. Blood dyscrasias and their management
5. Management of cardiac patient in the dentistry
6. Metabolic and endocrine disturbances, their oral manifestations
7. Nutritional deficiencies and their significance in dentistry
8. Oral sepsis and its effect on general system
9. Dysfunction of Temporomandibular joints
10. Cervicofacial lymphadenopathy
11. Diseases of salivary glands
12. Facial pain
13. Cysts and tumors of the oral cavity
14. Oral manifestations of dermatological and other systemic disturbances
15. Study of the influence of stress and psychosomatic factors in the treatment of dental diseases
16. Basic principles of immunology.

SCHEME OF EXAMINATION

Theory

Theory – 70 Marks
Viva Voce – 10 Marks
Internal Assessment (Theory) – 20 Marks

Oral Medicine and Radiology (Part-A + Part-B / 35 + 35 = 70)

Subject	*Type of question*	*Marks offered*	*Total*
Part-A/Oral Medicine and Forensic dentistry	Long essays	9	1 x 9 = 09
	Short notes	4	4 x 4 = 16
	Brief notes	2	5 x 2 = 10
Part-B/Oral Radiology	Long essays	9	1 x 9 = 09
	Short notes	4	4 x 4 = 16
	Brief notes	2	5 x 2 = 10

Clinicals

Clinicals – 70 Marks
Viva Voce – 10 Marks
Internal Assessment (Clinicals) – 20 Marks

REFERENCE BOOK

Oral Medicine: Textbook of Oral Medicine – By Anil Govindrao Ghom

AUTHOR ABBREVIATION

Ghom: Anil Govindrao Ghom

Edition: 1st

QUESTION BANK ABBREVIATION

Question Bank

LE — Long essays
SN — Short notes
BN — Brief notes

University

NTRUHS — Nandamuri Taraka Rama Rao University of Health Sciences
NTRUHS-NR — NTRUHS–New Regulations
NTRUHS-OR — NTRUHS–Old Regulations

CONTENTS

Contd...

Contd...

ORAL MEDICINE

Ghom

1. Oral Medicine Terminology

Long essays

Short notes

Brief notes

2. Case History Taking and Clinical Examination

Long essays

Short notes

1. Vitality tests?	NTR-NR	2004 Apr	80
2. Midpalatal swelling?	NTR-NR	2004 Apr	
3. Clinical examination of ulcer?	NTR-OR	1997 Apr	70

Brief notes

3. Developmental Disturbances of Oral Cavity

Long essays

Short notes

1. Anodontia?	NTR-OR	1997 Apr	117
2. Dentinogenesis imperfecta?	NTR-NR	2001 Oct	126
3. Regional odontodysplasia?	NTR-OR	1997 Apr	128

Brief notes

4. Regressive Changes of Oral Cavity

Long essays

Short notes

1. Pink tooth?	NTR-OR	1997 Apr	450
2. Resorption of roots?	NTR-OR	1996 Apr	458

Brief notes

Ghom

5. Physical and Chemical Injuries of Oral Cavity

Long essays

Short notes

Brief notes

6. Halitosis of Oral Cavity

Long essays

Short notes

Brief notes

7. Diseases of the Lip

Long essays

Short notes

1. Angioedema?	NTR-OR	1994 Nov	340
2. Angioneurotic edema?	NTR-OR	2000 Apr	340

Brief notes

8. Diseases of the Tongue

Long essays

1. Enumerate the papillae that are part in the atrophic changes on the tongue. Name the various conditions causing such changes?	NTR-OR	1987 May	464

Short notes

1. Bald tongue?	NTR-OR	1997 Oct	
	NTR-OR	2001 Oct	
2. Hairy tongue?	NTR-OR	1994 May	476
3. Glossopyrosis?	NTR-OR	1994 Nov	480
4. Geographic tongue?	NTR-NR	2001 Oct	478
5. Benign migratory glossitis?	NTR-NR	2002 Oct	475
6. Differential diagnosis of smooth tongue?	NTR-NR	2001 Oct	
7. How do you manage a case of carcinoma of tongue?	NTR-OR	1989 Jul	482

Brief notes

1. Glossodynia?	NTR-NR	2004 May	480
2. Glossopyrosis and Glossodynia?	NTR-NR	2002 Apr	480

				Ghom

9. Diseases of Gingival and Periodontal Tissues

Long essays

Short notes

1.	ANUG?	NTR-OR	1994 Nov	509
2.	Acute necrotizing ulcerative gingivitis?	NTR-NR	2000 Apr	509
3.	Pregnancy tumor and gingivitis?	NTR-OR	1994 May	515
4.	Herpetic gingivostomatitis?	NTR-NR	2006 Oct	510
5.	Clinical features of acute herpetic gingivostomatitis?	NTR-NR	2004 Oct	510

Brief notes

1.	ANUG?	NTR-NR	2006 Apr	509
2.	Cancrum oris?	NTR-NR	2002 Oct	665
3.	Gingival hyperplasia?	NTR-NR	2006 Apr	514

10. Diseases of Pulp and Periapical Tissues

Long essays

1.	Enumerate periapical radiolucencies and radiopacities. How would you diagnose systemic diseases with periapical changes in radiographs?	NTR-NR	2004 Oct	

Short notes

1.	Lamina dura?	NTR-OR	1993 May	
2.	Radiolucent lesions of periapical region?	NTR-NR	2001 Oct	
3.	How do you manage pulpitis and periodontitis?	NTR-OR	1990 Jul	

Brief notes

11. Dental Caries and Cariology

Long essays

Short notes

Brief notes

12. Disorders of Salivary Glands

Long essays

1.	What are the functions of saliva? Enumerate the causes of xerostomia and add a note on its management?	NTR-NR	2004 Oct	565, 570
2.	Enumerate the clinical features and radiological features of functional disturbances of salivary glands?	NTR-OR	1990 Feb	507, 569

			Ghom
3. Describe the procedure for sialography of parotid gland?	NTR-OR	1997 Oct	593
	NTR-OR	2001 Oct	
4. Describe sialography in detail and write briefly on its significance in various salivary gland disorders?	NTR-NR	2005 Apr	593

Short notes

1. Sialography?	NTR-NR	2006 Oct	
2. Xerostomia?	NTR-OR	1997 Apr	150
	NTR-OR	2000 Apr	
	NTR-NR	2001 Oct	
3. Sialolithiasis?	NTR-OR	1993 May	572
	NTR-NR	2002 Apr	
4. Sialometaplasia?	NTR-NR	2001 Oct	592
5. Necrotizing sialometaplasia?	NTR-OR	1999 Apr	592
6. Sjögren's syndrome?	NTR-OR	1993 May	581
	NTR-OR	2001 Apr	
	NTR-NR	2005 Apr	

Brief notes

1. Mucocele?	NTR-NR	2006 Oct	575

13. Disorders of Maxillary Sinus

Long essays

Short notes

1. Maxillary sinusitis?	NTR-OR	1994 Nov	498

Brief notes

14. Pigmented Lesions of Oral Cavity

Long essays

1. Discuss the differential diagnosis of oral mucosal pigmentation?	NTR-OR	1998 Apr	428

Short notes

1. Endogenous pigmentation?	NTR-NR	2006 Apr	427
2. Oral mucosal pigmentations?	NTR-OR	2000 Apr	427
3. Intrinsic stains and extrinsic stains?	NTR-OR	1990 Feb	
4. Pigmented lesions of orofacial pain?	NTR-OR	2004 Oct	427

Brief notes

Ghom

15. Premalignant Lesions and Conditions

Long essays

1. Enumerable premalignant conditions and lesions of oral mucosa. Describe in detail of any two of them?	NTR-OR	1997 Oct	155, 169
2. Enumerate premalignant conditions and premalignant lesions of oral mucosa, describe in detail any two of them?	NTR-OR	2001 Oct	155
3. Describe the clinical varieties of Leukoplakia and mention the treatment of different types of Leukoplakia. Add a note on etiology of Leukoplakia?	NTR-NR	2001 Apr	155
4. Classify white lesions of the oral cavity. Describe the etiology, clinical features, diagnosis and management of lichen planus?	NTR-OR	1999 Oct	155, 169
5. Classify the white lesions of the mouth describe in detail the clinical features differential diagnosis and managements of oral Lichenplanus?	NTR-OR	1991 Mar	155, 169
6. Describe the clinical features and management of oral submucous fibrosis. Discuss the etiological factors of this condition?	NTR-OR	1989 Jul	179
7. Enumerate premalignant lesions and premalignant conditions. Describe the etiology, clinical features and treatment of oral submucous fibrosis?	NTR-NR	2006 Apr	155
8. Describe the clinical features and management of a. Oral leukoplakia? b. Oral submucous fibrosis?	NTR-OR	1990 Jul	155

Short notes

1. Oral precancerous lesions?	NTR-OR	1994 May	155
	NTR-NR	2004 Oct	
2. Erythroplakia?	NTR-OR	1999 Oct	160
3. Speckled leukoplakia?	NTR-OR	1994 Nov	162
4. Leukoplakia treatment?	NTR-OR	2002 Apr	162
5. Treatment plan of leukoplakia?	NTR-OR	1993 May	162
6. Write briefly the identification and management of Leukoplakia?	NTR-OR	1990 Jul	162
7. How do you manage the speckled leukoplakia and Erosive lichen planus?	NTR-OR	1990 Jul	
8. Lichen planus?	NTR-OR	1998 Oct	178
9. Lichenoid reaction?	NTR-OR	2001 Oct	171
10. Diagnosis of oral lichen planus?	NTR-OR	1995 Apr	179
11. Submucous fibrosis?	NTR-OR	1993 May	
	NTR-OR	1998 Apr	183
	NTR-NR	2001 Oct	

			Ghom
12. Management of submucous fibrosis?	NTR-OR	1994 Nov	183
13. Enumerate the important differences between the submucous fibrosis and Scleroderma?	NTR-OR	1990 Feb	

Brief notes

1. Erosive lichenplanus?	NTR-NR	2005 Apr	171
2. Atrophic lichenplanus?	NTR-NR	2002 Oct	171
3. Management of submucosis fibrosis?	NTR-NR	2005 Apr	171

16. Red and White Lesions of the Oral Cavity

Long essays

1. Give the differential diagnosis of psoriasis?	NTR-OR	1989 Jul	
2. Enumerate the white lesions of the oral mucosa. Write about etiology, clinical features, investigations and management of oral thrush?	NTR-OR	2000 Apr	133, 139

Short notes

1. White sponge nevus?	NTR-OR	1997 Apr	149
2. Thrush?	NTR-OR	1997 Oct	139
	NTR-OR	1999 Apr	
3. Atrophic candidiasis?	NTR-OR	1999 Oct	141
4. Describe the clinical features and management of oral moniliasis?	NTR-OR	1990 Jul	139
5. Enumerate the important differences between the – Auspitz's sign and Tzanck test?	NTR-OR	1990 Feb	

Brief notes

1. Candidiasis?	NTR-NR	2006 Apr	139
2. Auspitz's sign?	NTR-NR	2002 Apr	148
3. White spongy nauves?	NTR-NR	2004 Apr	149

17. Vesicular and Bullous Lesions of the Oral Cavity

Long essays

1. Classify vesiculobullous lesions of oral cavity and site in detail about erythema multiforme?	NTR-OR	1998 Oct	336, 344
2. Enumerable various vesiculobullous lesion of oral cavity, describe erythema multiforme in detail?	NTR-OR	2001 Apr	336, 344
3. Classify the vesiculobullous lesions of oral caving. Add a note on the monogamist of oral mucous membrane pemphigoid?	NTR-OR	1991 Mar	336, 349
4. Classify vesiculobullous lesions. Discuss in detail Etiopathogenesis, clinical features and management of pemphigus vulgaris?	NTR-NR	2006 Oct	336, 349

			Ghom

Short notes

Question	Exam	Date	Ghom
1. Nikolsky's sign?	NTR-OR	1994 May	344
	NTR-OR	1996 Apr	
2. Erythema multiforme?	NTR-OR	1997 Oct	344
	NTR-OR	1999 Oct	
	NTR-OR	2001 Oct	
	NTR-NR	2002 Apr	
3. Stevens-Johnson syndrome?	NTR-NR	2000 Apr	345
	NTR-NR	2004 Apr	
4. Investigations with the result of pemphigus vulgaris?	NTR-OR	2005 Apr	348
5. How do you manage the pemphigus and pemphigoid?	NTR-OR	1990 Jul	348
6. Describe the oral manifestations of pemphigus vulgaris?	NTR-OR	1989 Jul	345
7. Describe briefly the classification and management of vesiculobullous lesions of the mouth?	NTR-OR	1990 Feb	336

Brief notes

18. Ulcerative and Erosive Lesions of the Oral Cavity

Long essays

Question	Exam	Date	Ghom
1. Discuss the differential diagnosis of multiple ulcers of oral mucosa?	NTR-NR	2000 Apr	338
2. Classify ulcers of the oral mucosa. Discuss the differential diagnosis of recurrent multiple ulcer?	NTR-OR	1999 Apr	336

Short notes

Question	Exam	Date	Ghom
1. Recurrent aphthous stomatitis?	NTR-OR	1997 Oct	341
2. Management of recurrent aphthous ulcers?	NTR-NR	2004 Oct	342

Brief notes

19. Disorders of Bones Manifested in the Jaws

Long essays

Question	Exam	Date	Ghom
1. Enumerate the clinical features and radiological features of a. Fibrous dysplasia? b. Radiopaque lesions of the jawbone? c. Chronic osteomyelitis at the angle of the mandible?	NTR-OR	1990 Feb	

Short notes

Question	Exam	Date	Ghom
1. Cherubism?	NTR-OR	1993 May	731
2. Fibrous dysplasia?	NTR-OR	1996 Apr	726
	NTR-OR	2001 Apr	

			Ghom
3. Describe the radiographic features of fibrous dysplasia?	NTR-OR	1989 Jul	727
4. Garre's osteomyelitis?	NTR-OR	2001 Apr	410
5. Condensing osteitis?	NTR-OR	1993 May	410
6. Osteoradionecrosis?	NTR-OR	1991 Mar	411
	NTR-OR	1994 May	
	NTR-OR	1999 Oct	
7. Describe the role of osteoradionecrosis in intraoral carinogenesis?	NTR-OR	1991 Mar	

Brief notes

1. Write briefly the osteomyelitis of mandible?	NTR-OR	1990 Jul	408
2. Radiographic appearance of Paget's disease?	NTR-NR	2002 Oct	737
3. Radiographic appearance of fibrous dysplasia?	NTR-NR	2006 Apr	736

20. TMJ Disorders

Long essays

1. What conditions may produce trismus. Describe in detail the predisposing factors, clinical features, treatment of oral submucous fibrosis?	NTR-OR	1989 Jan	391, 179
	NTR-OR	1993 Aug	
	NTR-OR	1994 Sep	
	NTR-OR	1996 Sep	

Short notes

1. Treatment of pericoronitis with trismus?	NTR-OR	1996 Apr	393

Brief notes

1. Trismus?	NTR-NR	2002 Apr	931

21. Orofacial Pain

Long essays

1. Give the differential diagnosis of pain in and around the tooth?	NTR-OR	1995 Apr	362
2. Describe the "pain in and around the tooth". Mention the treatment?	NTR-NR	2002 Apr	362
3. Discuss neuralgias affecting maxillofacial region. How would you treat Trigeminal neuralgias?	NTR-OR	1994 May	362, 370
4. Classify facial pain. Describe etiopathogenesis clinical features, and management of trigeminal neuralgia?	NTR-OR	1999 Oct	362, 370
5. Classify facial pain. Describe in detail etiology, clinical features and management of idiopathic trigeminal neuralgia?	NTR-OR	1997 Apr	362, 370

Short notes

Question	Exam	Year	Page
1. Classify the neuralgias in orofacial origin?	NTR-OR	1991 Mar	362
2. Subauricular pain?	NTR-NR	2001 Apr	
3. Atypical facial pain?	NTR-OR	1998 Apr	392
	NTR-OR	1999 Apr	
4. Atypical facial neuralgia?	NTR-OR	1995 Apr	369
5. Trigeminal neuralgia?	NTR-OR	1998 Oct	370
	NTR-NR	2006 Oct	
6. Management of Tic Douloureux?	NTR-NR	2006 Apr	372
7. Treatment of trigeminal neuralgia?	NTR-OR	1994 Nov	372
	NTR-NR	2001 Apr	
8. Management of trigeminal neuralgia?	NTR-OR	1996 Apr	372
9. How do you manage a case of trigeminal neuralgia?	NTR-OR	1989 Jul	372
10. Describe briefly the classification and management trigeminal neuralgia?	NTR-OR	1990 Feb	372
11. MPD syndrome?	NTR-OR	2000 Apr	555
12. Myofacial pain dysfunction syndrome?	NTR-OR	1991 Mar	555
	NTR-NR	2004 May	
	NTR-OR	2004 Oct	
13. Burning mouth syndrome?	NTR-OR	1999 Apr	375
	NTR-NR	2004 Apr	
14. Enumerate the important differences between the—paroxysmal neuralgias and atypical neuralgias?	NTR-OR	1998 Oct	

Brief notes

Question	Exam	Year	Page
1. Bell's palsy?	NTR-NR	2006 Apr	707
2. Myofacial pain dysfunction syndrome?	NTR-OR	1990 Feb	555
3. Management of paroxysmal trigeminal neuralgia?	NTR-NR	2004 Oct	372

22. Trauma to Teeth and Facial Structures

Long essays

Short notes

Brief notes

23. Odontogenic Cysts and Tumors

Long essays

Short notes

Question	Exam	Year	Page
1. Dentigerous cyst?	NTR-OR	1993 May	234
	NTR-OR	1994 May	
2. Ameloblastoma?	NTR-NR	2002 Oct	236
3. Radiographic appearance of ameloblastoma?	NTR-OR	1998 Oct	236

			Ghom
4. Describe the radiographic features of ameloblastoma?	NTR-OR	1989 Jul	236
	NTR-OR	1993 May	
5. Odontogenic Keratocyst?	NTR-OR	1998 Apr	197
6. Radiographic appearance of odontogenic keratocyst?	NTR-NR	2004 Oct	198

Brief notes

1. Radiographic appearance of periapical cemental dysplasia?	NTR-NR	2005 Apr	243

24. Non-Odontogenic Cysts and Tumors

Long essays

Short notes

Brief notes

25. Benign Tumors of the Oral Cavity

Long essays

Short notes

1. Myxoma?	NTR-OR	1994 May	260
2. Pleomorphic adenoma of palate?	NTR-OR	1995 Apr	289
3. Ossifying fibroma—clinical features?	NTR-NR	2002 Apr	739
4. Describe the radiographic features of Myxoma?	NTR-OR	1989 Jul	260

Brief notes

26. Malignant Tumors of the Oral Cavity

Long essays

1. Describe the clinical features and management of oral cancers?	NTR-OR	1990 Jul	

Short notes

1. Kaposi's sarcoma?	NTR-OR	1999 Apr	429
2. Oral cancer—predisposing factors?	NTR-NR	2001 Apr	287

Brief notes

27. Diseases of Respiratory Tract

Long essays

Short notes

Brief notes

Ghom

28. Diseases of Cardiovascular System

Long essays

Short notes

Brief notes

29. Diseases of Gastrointestinal Tract

Long essays

Short notes

Brief notes

30. Diseases of Renal System

Long essays

Short notes

Brief notes

31. Hematological Disorders

Long essays

1. Define and classify anemias. Discuss in detail about iron deficiency anemia?	NTR-NR	2002 Oct	793
2. Enumerate the causes of cervical lymphadenopathy and give the clinical features of Hodgkin's diseases?	NTR-NR	2005 Apr	313
3. Classify bleeding disorders of the mouse. How do you manage a case of myeloid race leukemia patient visiting dental hospital?	NTR-OR	1991 Mar	318

Short notes

1. Agranulocytosis?	NTR-OR	1999 Apr	700
	NTR-NR	2001 Apr	
2. Cyclic neutropenia?	NTR-OR	1999 Oct	800
	NTR-NR	2001 Oct	
3. Thalassemia major?	NTR-OR	1998 Oct	790
4. Eosinophilic granuloma?	NTR-NR	2001 Apr	835
5. Chronic lymphatic leukemia?	NTR-NR	2002 Oct	322
6. Sideropenic dysphagia?	NTR-OR	2000 Apr	
7. Oral manifestations of anemia?	NTR-NR	2006 Oct	795
8. Clinical features of pernicious anemia?	NTR-NR	2005 Apr	795
9. Describe briefly the classification and management of bleeding disorders of mouth?	NTR-OR	1990 Feb	

Ghom

Brief notes

1. Hodgkin's disease?	NTR-NR	2002 Oct	313

32. Endocrine Disorders

Long essays

1. Describe the oral manifestations of endocrine diseases?	NTR-NR	2004 May	771

Short notes

1. Hyperparathyroidism?	NTR-OR	1999 Apr	771
	NTR-NR	2002 Oct	
2. Hyperparathyroidism – investigative?	NTR-NR	2002 Apr	771
3. Describe the oral manifestations of primary hyperparathyroidism?	NTR-OR	1989 Jul	771
4. Oral manifestations of diabetes mellitus?	NTR-NR	2006 Apr	774
5. Describe the oral manifestations of diabetes mellitus?	NTR-OR	1989 Jul	774
6. Oral manifestations and dental considerations in diabetic mellitus?	NTR-NR	2004 Sep	774

Brief notes

1. Hyperparathyroidism?	NTR-NR	2002 Oct	771

33. Neuromuscular Disorders

Long essays

Short notes

Brief notes

34. Allergic and Immunological Diseases

Long essays

Short notes

Brief notes

35. Infections of Oral Cavity and Oral Sepsis

Long essays

1. Define social sepsis? Describe its local and systemic effect?	NTR-OR	1993 May	424
2. Describe the oral manifestations of secondary infected syphilis?	NTR-OR	1987 May	643

Ghom

Short notes

1.	Mumps?	NTR-OR	1998 Apr	577
2.	Hutchinson's triad?	NTR-OR	2001 Oct	643
3.	Serological test for syphilis?	NTR-OR	2001 Apr	673
4.	Herpes zoster?	NTR-NR	2002 Oct	667
5.	Herpes labialis?	NTR-NR	2002 Oct	667
6.	Herpes stomatitis?	NTR-OR	1996 Apr	517
7.	How do you manage herpangina and Herpetic stomatitis?	NTR-OR	1990 Jul	517
8.	How do you manage a case of herpetic stomatitis?	NTR-OR	1989 Jul	670
9.	Describe briefly the classification and management of acute infections of the oral cavity?	NTR-OR	1990 Feb	389

Brief notes

1.	Secondary stage of syphilis?	NTR-NR	2002 Oct	643

36. Acquired Immunodeficiency Syndrome

Long essays

Short notes

1.	Hairy leukoplakia?	NTR-NR	2001 Apr	758
2.	Oral manifestations of HIV infection?	NTR-OR	2004 Oct	756

Brief notes

1.	HIV?	NTR-NR	2004 Apr	752
2.	Hairy leukoplakia?	NTR-NR	2006 Oct	758

37. Infection Control in Dentistry

Long essays

Short notes

Brief notes

38. Diagnostic Aids in Dentistry

Long essays

1. Enumerate the importance of the
   a. Intravital staining?
   b. Peripheral blood picture in oral medicine?
   c. Role of immunoglobulin in oral medicine?
   d. Bisecting techniques of intraoral radiographs? NTR-OR 1983 Jul

Short notes

1. Biopsy?	NTR-OR	1996 Apr	76
	NTR-OR	1997 Oct	
	NTR-OR	1999 Apr	
	NTR-OR	2000 Apr	
	NTR-NR	2000 Apr	
2. Patch test?	NTR-OR	1994 Nov	
3. Paget's test?	NTR-OR	1999 Oct	
4. Schimmer's test?	NTR-OR	1999 Oct	
5. Rose Waller test?	NTR-NR	2004 Oct	
6. Paul-Bunnel test?	NTR-NR	2006 Apr	
7. Exfoliative cytology?	NTR-OR	1997 Apr	79
	NTR-OR	1998 Apr	
8. Oral exfoliative cytology?	NTR-OR	1998 Oct	
9. Role of intravital staining in oral medicine?	NTR-OR	1991 Mar	
10. Describe the role of peripheral blood smear in oral medicine?	NTR-OR	1991 Mar	

Brief notes

1. Patch test?	NTR-NR	2002 Apr	

39. Pharmacotherapy in Dentistry

Long essays

1. Describe the merits and demerits of using corticosteroids in oral lesions with suitable examples?	NTR-OR	1994 Nov	

Short notes

1. Antiviral drugs?	NTR-OR	1999 Apr	873
2. Antifungal drugs?	NTR-OR	2000 Apr	861
3. Anti-inflammatory drugs?	NTR-OR	2001 Apr	854
4. Corticosteroids in dentistry?	NTR-OR	1998 Oct	
5. Antibiotics in oral diseases?	NTR-OR	1991 Mar	850
6. 17 Ketosteroids in oral medicine?	NTR-OR	1991 Mar	

Brief notes

1. Role of antibiotic therapy?	NTR-OR	1990 Feb	

40. Lasers in Dental Practice

Long essays

Short notes

Brief notes

Ghom

41. Computers in Dental Practice

Long essays

Short notes

Brief notes

42. Medical Problems in Dentistry

Long essays

Short notes

1. Pregnancy, gingivitis and tumor?	NTR-OR	1994 May	283
2. Management of cardiac patient in dental extraction?	NTR-NR	2004 Apr	

Brief notes

1. Syncope?	NTR-OR	1990 Jul	724
2. Anaphylactic shock?	NTR-NR	2005 Apr	851
3. Precautions to be taken during dental treatment of cardiac patient?	NTR-NR	2006 Oct	

43. Professional Hazards in Dentistry

Long essays

Short notes

Brief notes

44. Nutritional and Metabolic Disorders

Long essays

1. Describe the oral aspects of Hypovitaminosis?	NTR-OR	1994 Nov	813

Short notes

1. Avitaminosis-A?	NTR-NR	2001 Apr	

Brief notes

45. Syndromes of the Oral Cavity

Long essays

Short notes

1. Eagle's syndrome?	NTR-OR	1997 Apr	902
	NTR-OR	1998 Oct	
2. Trotter's syndrome?	NTR-NR	2000 Apr	909
	NTR-NR	2001 Apr	

			Ghom
3. Sjögren's syndrome?	NTR-NR	2005 Apr	909
4. Grinspan syndrome?	NTR-OR	1997 Apr	
5. Hereford's syndrome?	NTR-OR	1998 Apr	904
6. Ramsay Hunt syndrome?	NTR-OR	1995 Apr	908
	NTR-OR	1997 Oct	
	NTR-OR	1999 Apr	
	NTR-OR	2001 Oct	
7. Burning mouth syndrome?	NTR-OR	1999 Apr	900
	NTR-NR	2000 Apr	
8. Plummer Vinson's syndrome?	NTR-OR	1994 May	
9. Steven Johnson's syndrome?	NTR-NR	2000 Apr	909
	NTR-NR	2004 Apr	
10. Melkerson Rosenthal syndrome?	NTR-OR	1998 Apr	906
11. Myofacial pain dysfunction syndrome?	NTR-NR	2004 Apr	907
Brief notes			
1. Eagle's syndrome?	NTR-NR	2005 Apr	902
	NTR-NR	2006 Oct	
2. Battered baby syndrome?	NTR-NR	2006 Apr	

46. Transplantation Medicine

Long essays

Short notes

Brief notes

47. Geriatrics and Oral Medicine

Long essays

Short notes

Brief notes

48. Occupational Hazards in Dentistry

Long essays

Short notes

Brief notes

49. Biopsychomodel of Illness and Oral Medicine

Long essays

Short notes

			Ghom

Brief notes

1. Phsychogenic disease?	NTR-NR	2001 Oct	

50. Miscellaneous Topics

Long essays

1. Give the differential diagnosis of swelling in the midline of the palate?	NTR-OR	1996 Apr	
2. Write the definitions of various basic lesions of oral mucosa. Write the names of three diseases for each of the basic lesion?	NTR-NR	2001 Oct	

Short notes

1. Dysgeusia?	NTR-OR	1997 Oct	
	NTR-OR	2001 Oct	
2. Id reaction?	NTR-OR	1998 Oct	
3. Auspitz's sign?	NTR-NR	2002 Apr	942
4. Nikolsky's sign?	NTR-OR	1994 May	942
	NTR-OR	1996 Apr	
5. Mucus patches?	NTR-OR	1998 Apr	645
6. Metallic stomatitis?	NTR-OR	1987 Mar	
7. Stomatitis veneneta?	NTR-OR	1996 Apr	
	NTR-NR	2004 Apr	
8. Mid palatal swelling?	NTR-NR	2004 Apr	
9. Sideropenic dysphagia?	NTR-NR	2000 Apr	
10. Hormone dependent gums?	NTR-OR	1990 Feb	
11. Control of bleeding?	NTR-OR	1994 May	
12. Periapical osteofibrosis?	NTR-OR	1994 May	
13. Importance of asking DLC?	NTR-OR	1994 May	
14. Various types of periosteal reactions in sarcoma?	NTR-OR	1987 May	942

Brief notes

1. Red teeth?	NTR-NR	2002 Apr	
2. T-lymphocytes?	NTR-NR	2002 Apr	
3. Epithelial dysplasia?	NTR-NR	2002 Apr	
4. Stony hard lymph node?	NTR-NR	2004 Apr	
5. Cleidocranial dysostosis?	NTR-NR	2005 Apr	105

ORAL RADIOLOGY

SYLLABUS

1. Physics of radiation and properties of X-rays.
2. Principles of X-ray techniques and factors for radiography and fluoroscopy.
3. Technique of intra-oral and extra-oral radiography and normal anatomical land marks.
4. Radiological interpretations of abnormal dental and jaw conditions.
5. Elements of radiation treatment in oral and facial conditions and their sequelae.
6. Contrast radiography and recent advances in dental radiology including radio-active isotopes.
7. Protection measures of radiation in dental X-ray laboratories.
8. Biological effects of radiation.

SCHEME OF EXAMINATION

Theory

Theory	–	70 Marks
Viva Voce	–	10 Marks
Internal Assessment (Theory)	–	20 Marks

Oral Medicine and Radiology (Part-A + Part-B / 35 + 35 = 70)

Subject	*Type of question*	*Marks offered*	*Total*
Part-A/Oral Medicine and Forensic Dentistry	Long essays	9	1 x 9 = 09
	Short notes	4	4 x 4 = 16
	Brief notes	2	5 x 2 = 10
Part-B/Oral Radiology	Long essays	9	1 x 9 = 09
	Short notes	4	4 x 4 = 16
	Brief notes	2	5 x 2 = 10

Clinicals

Clinicals	–	70 Marks
Viva Voce	–	10 Marks
Internal Assessment (Clinicals)	–	20 Marks

REFERENCE BOOK

Oral Radiology: Essentials of Oral Radiology – By Pramod John

AUTHOR ABBREVIATION

John: Pramod John

Edition: 1st

QUESTION BANK ABBREVIATION

Question Bank

LE — Long essays
SN — Short notes
BN — Brief notes

University

NTRUHS — Nandamuri Taraka Rama Rao University of Health Sciences
NTRUHS-NR — NTRUHS–New Regulations
NTRUHS-OR — NTRUHS–Old Regulations

CONTENTS

Contd...

Contd...

ORAL RADIOLOGY

John

1. History of Radiology

Long essays

Short notes

1. Radiology and Roentology?	NTR-OR	2001 Oct	2

Brief notes

2. Radiation Physics

Long essays

Short notes

1. Dosimetry?	NTR-OR	1998 Oct	36

Brief notes

3. Properties of X-rays

Long essays

Short notes

1. Properties of X-rays	NTR-OR	1998 Apr	12

Brief notes

1. Properties of X-rays?	NTR-NR	2006 Oct	12

4. Production of X-rays

Long essays

Short notes

1. Collimeters?	NTR-OR	1997 Apr	24
2. Collimation?	NTR-NR	2002 Oct	23
3. X-ray tube?	NTR-OR	1997 Oct	13
	NTR-NR	2001 Oct	
4. Colidge tube?	NTR-OR	1998 Apr	
5. Filters and Collimeters?	NTR-OR	1993 May	23
6. Characteristic radiation?	NTR-OR	1999 Apr	21

John

7. Collimation and filtration?	NTR-OR	2001 Apr	23
8. Generation of X-rays?	NTR-NR	2005 Apr	20

Brief notes

1. Filters and collimation in radiography?	NTR-OR	1987 May	23
2. Thermoluminescent dosimeter?	NTR-NR	2006 Apr	36

5. Radiation Biology

Long essays

1. Describe in detail the radiation hazards in Orofacial region and mention its preventive measures?	NTR-OR	1993 May	35, 38
2. Discuss briefly radiation hazards. Describe the various methods to protect the patient and operator from the hazards?	NTR-OR	2001 Apr	33, 38
3. Enumerate hazards of radiation. Discuss the effects of radiation on oral tissues?	NTR-OR	2000 Apr	33, 35

Short notes

1. Osteoradionecrosis?	NTR-OR	1991 Mar	
	NTR-OR	1999 Oct	
2. Radiation caries?	NTR-OR	1998 Oct	130
	NTR-NR	2000 Apr	
	NTR-OR	2001 Oct	
3. Radiation hazards of jaws?	NTR-NR	2002 Apr	36
4. Hazards of radiation?	NTR-NR	2006 Apr	33
5. Radiation hazards of teeth, oral mucosa and the jaws?	NTR-NR	2004 Oct	35

Brief notes

6. Protection from Radiation

Long essays

1. Discuss in detail regarding radiation protection?	NTR-NR	2002 Oct	38
2. Describe in detail the radiation hazards in Orofacial region and mention its preventive measures?	NTR-OR	1993 May	33, 38
3. Discuss briefly radiation hazards. Describe the various methods to protect the patient and operator from the hazards?	NTR-OR	2001 Apr	38, 38
4. Enumerate various techniques of taking intraoral radiography. Discuss in detail the various procedures taken to protect the operator and the patient during radiography?	NTR-NR	2006 Oct	75, 38

John

Short notes

1. Radiation protection?	NTR-OR	1994 May	38
2. Radiation protection for patient?	NTR-NR	2005 Apr	39
3. Radiation protection of operator?	NTR-OR	1999 Apr	40

Brief notes

7. Ideal Radiograph

Long essays

Short notes

Brief notes

8. Faulty Radiograph

Long essays

1. Discuss "Faulty IO radiographs".	NTR-NR	2002 Apr	68
2. Discuss the causes of faulty radiographs.	NTR-OR	1998 Oct	68

Short notes

Brief notes

9. X-ray Film, Intensifying Screens and Grids

Long essays

1. Composition of intraoral periapical films?	NTR-OR	2001 Apr	42

Short notes

1. Grids?	NTR-OR	1998 Apr	47
	NTR-OR	2000 Apr	
	NTR-NR	2000 Apr	
	NTR-OR	2001 Oct	
	NTR-NR	2002 Oct	
2. Radiographic film?	NTR-OR	1999 Apr	42
3. X-ray film?	NTR-OR	1995 Apr	42
4. X-ray film pocket?	NTR-NR	2001 Oct	44
5. Radiographic films?	NTR-NR	2002 Oct	42
6. Potter bucky diaphragm	NTR-OR	2001 Oct	105
7. Composition of intra-oral periapical film?	NTR-OR	2001 Apr	42
8. Occlusal film?	NTR-OR	1996 Apr	45
9. Occlusal radiograph?	NTR-OR	2000 Apr	45
10. Indications of occlusal films?	NTR-NR	2006 Apr	45
11. Intensifying screen?	NTR-OR	1994 Nov	50
	NTR-OR	1996 Apr	

			John
	NTR-OR	1997 Apr	
	NTR-OR	1998 Oct	
	NTR-OR	1999 Oct	
	NTR-OR	2001 Apr	
	NTR-NR	2001 Apr	
	NTR-NR	2005 Apr	

Brief notes

1. Grid?	NTR-NR	2005 Apr	104
2. Potter bucky diaphragm	NTR-NR	2004 Oct	105

10. Process of X-ray Film

Long essays

1. What is the composition of radiographic film? Describe the mechanism of image formation. Add a note on the composition of developing and fixing solution and their functions?	NTR-NR	2006 Apr	42, 55

Short notes

1. Occlusal film?	NTR-OR	1996 Apr	45
2. Composition of fixer?	NTR-OR	2001 Oct	58
3. X-ray fixing solution?	NTR-OR	1994 May	58
4. Automatic film processing?	NTR-NR	2006 Apr	63
5. Processing of X-ray film?	NTR-NR	2002 Oct	59
6. Processing of an intraoral film?	NTR-OR	1993 May	59
7. Requirements of dark room?	NTR-NR	2001 Oct	60
8. Composition and action of fixer solution?	NTR-OR	2000 Apr	58
9. Contents and action of developing and fixing solution?	NTR-OR	1997 Oct	56
	NTR-OR	2001 Apr	

Brief notes

11. Radiographic Quality Assurance and Infection

Long essays

Short notes

Brief notes

12. Normal Radiographic Anatomy

Long essays

Short notes

1. Lamina dura?	NTR-OR	1993 May	83
2. Radiopaque lesions of the jawbones?	NTR-OR	1991 Mar	84
3. Describe the radiopaque lesions of the jawbones?	NTR-OR	1990 Feb	84

Brief notes

13. Projection Geometry

Long essays

1. Enumerate intraoral radiographic technique. Describe the procedure of localizing an impacted left maxillary canine?	NTR-OR	1999 Apr	75

Short notes

1. Target film distance?	NTR-NR	2002 Apr	

Brief notes

14. Intraoral Radiographic Examination

Long essays

1. Describe the angulations for full-mouth periapical radiographs?	NTR-OR	1987 May	75
2. How will you take intraoral radiograph of upper permanent molar?	NTR-OR	1995 Apr	74
3. Describe the procedure of periapical radiograph of the mandibular central incisor using short cone technique?	NTR-OR	1998 Apr	
4. Compare bisecting angle short cone technique and long cones technique of radiography. Describe technique of lower third molar?	NTR-OR	1994 May	
5. What are the various factors affecting the dental radiographs? Describe in detail the placement of film in periapical intraoral radiography.	NTR-OR	1996 Apr	

Short notes

1. Long cone technique?	NTR-NR	2001 Apr	
2. Occlusal radiograph	NTR-OR	2001 Apr	78
3. Occlusal view radiography?	NTR-NR	2002 Oct	78
4. Bitewing radiograph?	NTR-OR	2000 Apr	78
	NTR-NR	2000 Apr	

5. Indications of bitewing radiography?	NTR-NR	2006 Oct	78
6. Angulation of upper molar?	NTR-OR	2001 Oct	
7. Indications of transorbital view?	NTR-NR	2004 Oct	76
8. Enumerate the importance of bisecting techniques of intraoral radiographs?	NTR-OR	1990 Feb	78

Brief notes

15. Extraoral Radiographic Examination

Long essays

1. How will you take lateral oblique view of mandible and give interpretations to that?	NTR-OR	1989 Jul	91

Short notes

1. PA view radiograph?	NTR-OR	1999 Apr	94
2. Submentovertex view?	NTR-NR	2005 Apr	96

Brief notes

1. Indications of PA view skull?	NTR-NR	2006 Oct	96

16. Panoramic Imaging

Long essays

Short notes

1. Orthopantomograph?	NTR-OR	1997 Oct	94
2. Pan oral radiography?	NTR-OR	1994 May	96

Brief notes

17. Digital Imaging

Long essays

Short notes

Brief notes

18. Specialized Radiographic Techniques

Long essays

Short notes

1. Contrast radiography?	NTR-OR	2001 Apr	
2. Magnetic resonance image?	NTR-OR	1996 Apr	121

Brief notes

19. Guidelines for Prescribing Dental Radiographs

Long essays

Short notes

Brief notes

20. Principles of Radiographic Interpretations

Long essays

Short notes

Brief notes

21. Dental Caries

Long essays

Short notes

1. Radiation caries?	NTR-OR	1998 Oct	130
	NTR-NR	2000 Apr	
	NTR-OR	2001 Oct	
2. Radiological appearance of dental caries?	NTR-OR	1997 Oct	125

Brief notes

22. Periodontal Diseases

Long essays

Short notes

1. Radiographic appearance of periapical cemental dysplasia?	NTR-NR	2005 Apr	184

Brief notes

23. Dental Anomalies

Long essays

Short notes

Brief notes

John

24. Inflammatory Lesions of Oral Cavity

Long essays

1. Enumerate the periapical radiolucencies and radiopacities. How would you diagnose systemic diseases with periapical changes in radiographs?	NTR-NR	2004 Oct	189

Short notes

1. Radiolucent lesions of periapical region?	NTR-NR	2001 Oct	

Brief notes

25. Cysts of the Jaws

Long essays

1. Describe the radiographic appearance of different cysts of maxilla and mandible?	NTR-NR	2001 Apr	158

Short notes

1. Radiographic appearance of odontogenic keratocyst?	NTR-NR	2004 Oct	161

Brief notes

26. Benign Tumors of the Jaws

Long essays

Short notes

1. Radiographic appearance of ameloblastoma?	NTR-OR	1993 May	166
	NTR-OR	1998 Oct	
2. Describe the radiographic appearance of Myxoma?	NTR-OR	1989 Jul	
3. Describe the radiographic appearance of ameloblastoma?	NTR-OR	1989 Jul	166

Brief notes

27. Malignant Diseases of the Jaws

Long essays

Short notes

Brief notes

28. Diseases of Bone Manifested in the Jaws

Long essays

1. Describe the radiographic appearance of different stages of osteomyelitis of jaws?	NTR-NR	2002 Apr	156

Short notes

1. Radiographic appearance of osteosarcoma?	NTR-OR	2000 Apr	
2. Radiographic appearance of Paget's disease?	NTR-NR	2002 Oct	187

Brief notes

1. Radiographic appearance of fibrous dysplasia?	NTR-NR	2006 Apr	182

29. Systemic Diseases Manifested in the Jaws

Long essays

Short notes

1. Describe the radiological appearance of fibrous dysplasia?	NTR-OR	1989 Jul	182

Brief notes

30. Diagnostic Imaging of the Temporomandibular Joint

Long essays

Short notes

1. Radiologic anatomy of temporomandibular joint?	NTR-OR	1994 May	213

Brief notes

31. Paranasal Sinuses

Long essays

1. Write the differential diagnosis of radiopacities of maxillary antrum?	NTR-OR	1987 May	

Short notes

Brief notes

32. Soft Tissue Calcification and Ossification

Long essays

Short notes

Brief notes

33. Trauma to Teeth and Facial Structures

Long essays

1. Enumerate the various radiographic techniques for the diagnosis of fracture of mandible?	NTR-NR	2000 Apr	144

John

Short notes

Brief notes

34. Developmental Disturbances of Face and Jaws

Long essays

Short notes

Brief notes

35. Salivary Gland Radiology

Long essays

1. Describe the procedure for sialography of parotid gland?	NTR-OR NTR-OR	1997 Oct 2001 Oct	117
2. Describe sialography in detail and write briefly on its significance in various salivary gland disorders?	NTR-NR	2005 Apr	117

Short notes

1. Sialography?	NTR-NR	2006 Oct	117

Brief notes

36. Orofacial Implants

Long essays

Short notes

Brief notes

37. Miscellaneous

Long essays

1. Discuss the differential diagnosis of radiolucencies on coronal part of the teeth?	NTR-OR	1999 Oct
2. Describe the five principles of image production in relation to periapical radiography?	NTR-NR	2001 Oct
3. Describe the differential diagnosis of radiolucent lesions in posterior part of the body of the mandible?	NTR-OR	1997 Apr

Short notes

1. Timer?	NTR-NR	2001 Apr
2. Angulation?	NTR-OR	1995 Apr
3. Compton effect?	NTR-OR	1998 Oct

			John
4. SLOB?	NTR-NR	2002 Oct	112
5. SLOB formula?	NTR-OR	1999 Oct	112
6. SLOB formula or principle?	NTR-NR	2001 Oct	112
7. ALARA?	NTR-NR	2000 Apr	112
8. Moth-eaten appearance	NTR-OR	2004 Oct	
9. Multilocular radiolucencies of jawbone?	NTR-OR	2006 Oct	

Brief notes

1. Resolution?	NTR-NR	2004 Oct
2. Sunray appearance?	NTR-NR	2006 Apr

ORAL AND MAXILLOFACIAL SURGERY

SYLLABUS

1. Impactions—classification of mandibular and maxillary impactions. Surgical management and associated complications
2. Maxillary sinus—surgical anatomy, surgical approach
3. Oro-antral fistula—clinical features and management
4. Emergencies in oral surgery—shock, syncope, electrolyte imbalance, hemorrhage and their management in oral surgery
5. Blood grouping and transfusion
6. Sterilization and asepsis
7. Infections of the oral cavity—anatomy of the facial spaces
8. Acute alveolar abscess, Ludwig's angina, cancrum oris
9. Inflammatory diseases of the jaw bones—osteomyelitis, its pathogenesis, treatment and complications
10. Benign cystic lesions of the jaws—definition, classifications, pathogenesis and diagnosis
11. Benign cystic lesions of the jaws—differential diagnosis
12. Benign cystic lesions and management
13. Neuralgias—Trigeminal neuralgia
14. Pre-prosthetic surgery I—Alveoplasty
15. Pre-prosthetic surgery II—Vestibuloplasty
16. Pre-prosthetic surgery III—Surgical aids to orthodontics
17. TMJ surgical anatomy, dislocation and subluxation etc
18. Trismus and ankylosis and other causes of inability to open the mouth and its treatment
19. Pain dysfunction syndrome
20. Fractures of the jaws: introduction, surgical anatomy of the mandible and classification of fractures
21. Clinical features, including radiological examination and preliminary management of maxillofacial injuries
22. Management of mandibular fractures, fractures at the body of the mandible
23. Angle fractures and edentulous fractures
24. Mandibular condylar fractures
25. Fractures of middle third of the face—classification and preliminary management
26. Management of middle third fractures
27. Fractures of zygomatic complex and management
28. Complications of the fractures
29. Odontogenic tumors—classification, ameloblastoma and odontomes, etc.
30. Tumors of the lip, tongue, mouth, jaws and salivary glands. Management with elementary knowledge of radiation therapy
31. Salivary glands—sialadenitis, sialogram, salivary calculi and management. Neoplasms arising from minor salivary glands
32. Developmental deformities—harelip, cleft lip and palate and developmental deformities of the jaws
33. Preservation of the infected teeth—apicoectomy, transplantation and Replantation, etc.
34. Cryosurgery—principles of cryosurgery and its applications in the treatment of oral lesions

SCHEME OF EXAMINATION

Theory

Theory	–	70 Marks
Viva Voce	–	10 Marks
Internal Assessment (Theory)	–	20 Marks

Oral Pathology (Part-A + Part-B / 35 + 35 = 70)

Subject	*Type of question*	*Marks offered*	*Total*
Part-A/Oral and Maxillofacial Surgery	Long essays	9	1 x 9 = 09
	Short notes	4	4 x 4 = 16
	Brief notes	2	5 x 2 = 10
Part-B/Oral and Maxillofacial Surgery	Long essays	9	1 x 9 = 09
	Short notes	4	4 x 4 = 16
	Brief notes	2	5 x 2 = 10

Clinicals

Clinicals	–	70 Marks
Viva Voce	–	10 Marks
Internal Assessment (Clinicals)	–	20 Marks

REFERENCE BOOK

Oral and Maxillofacial Surgery: Textbook of Oral Surgery – By Neelima Anil Malik

AUTHOR ABBREVIATION

Neelima: Neelima Anil Malik

Edition: 2nd

QUESTION BANK ABBREVIATION

Question Bank

LE — Long essays
SN — Short notes
BN — Brief notes

University

NTRUHS — Nandamuri Taraka Rama Rao University of Health Sciences
NTRUHS-NR — NTRUHS–New Regulations
NTRUHS-OR — NTRUHS–Old Regulations

CONTENTS

Contd...

Contd...

ORAL AND MAXILLOFACIAL SURGERY

Neelima

1. Scope and Objectives of Oral Surgery

Long essays

Short notes

Brief notes

2. Basic Principles of Oral Surgery

Long essays

Short notes

Brief notes

3. Decision Making in Oral Surgery

Long essays

Short notes

Brief notes

4. Ethics and Medicolegal Considerations

Long essays

Short notes

Brief notes

5. Clinical History and Physical Examination

Long essays

Short notes

Brief notes

6. Diagnostic AIDS in Oral Surgery

Long essays

Short notes

1. Biopsy?	NTR-OR	1993 May	17
	NTR-OR	1998 Apr	
	NTR-NR	2002 Oct	
2. Cephalometry?	NTR-NR	2002 Apr	270
3. Cephelometric analysis?	NTR-NR	2002 Oct	270
4. Cephalometry in oral surgery?	NTR-OR	2001 Oct	270
5. Biopsy Indications and diagnosis techniques?	NTR-NR	2002 Apr	17

Brief notes

1. Incisional biopsy?	NTR-NR	2006 Oct	17
2. Exfoliative cytology?	NTR-NR	2004 Apr	16

7. Essential Laboratory Investigations

Long essays

Short notes

Brief notes

8. Therapeutics in Oral Surgery

Long essays

Short notes

1. Aspirin	NTR-OR	1997 Apr	
2. Penicillins	NTR-OR	2000 Apr	106
3. Pentazocine	NTR-OR	1992 Nov	149
4. Premedication	NTR-OR	1992 Nov	147
	NTR-OR	1997 Apr	
	NTR-OR	1998 Apr	
	NTR-NR	2004 May	
	NTR-NR	2005 Apr	
5. Cephalosporines	NTR-OR	1999 Oct	107
6. Diclofenac sodium	NTR-OR	2000 Apr	
7. Anti-inflammatory drugs	NTR-NR	2001 Oct	
8. Analgesic in OMF surgery	NTR-NR	2002 Oct	149
9. Broad-spectrum penicillins?	NTR-OR	2001 Apr	102
10. Antibiotic for orofacial infection	NTR-NR	2004 Apr	102
11. Presurgical antibiotic prophylaxis	NTR-NR	2004 Oct	114
12. Principles of antibiotic therapy?	NTR-NR	2006 Oct	103

Brief notes

1. Diazepam	NTR-NR	2004 Oct	148
2. Idiosyncrasy?	NTR-NR	2002 Oct	
3. Chemotherapy?	NTR-NR	2004 Apr	147
4. Pre-medication	NTR-NR	2004 Apr	
	NTR-OR	1998 Apr	
5. Prophylactic antibiotic therapy?	NTR-NR	2005 Oct	114

9. Sterilization and Asepsis

Long essays

1. Define asepsis? What precaution would you take to maintain asepsis during a minor oral surgical procedure?	NTR-OR	1996 Apr	70

Short notes

1. Asepsis?	NTR-OR	1991 Oct	70
2. Sterilization	NTR-OR	1994 May	72
	NTR-NR	2002 Oct	
3. Moist heat sterilization	NTR-NR	2004 Oct	72

Brief notes

1. Sterilization?	NTR-NR	2005 Apr	72
2. Cold sterilization?	NTR-NR	2006 Oct	
3. Crossinfection in dental office?	NTR-NR	2004 Apr	87

10. Biomaterial Used in Oral and Maxillofacial Surgery

Long essays

Short notes

1. Bone plates?	NTR-OR	1989 Feb	395
2. Mucoperiosteal flaps?	NTR-OR	1997 Apr	120
3. Miniplate osteosynthesis?	NTR-OR	1999 Oct	395
4. Suture materials used in oral surgery	NTR-NR	2001 Oct	59
5. Suture material and suturing techniques	NTR-NR	2002 Oct	59
6. Name various flap designs used for minor oral surgery?	NTR-NR	2002 Apr	120

Brief notes

1. Suturing?	NTR-NR	2006 Oct	59
2. Types of mucoperiosteal flaps?	NTR-NR	2006 Oct	120

11. Armamentarium Used in Oral and Maxillofacial Surgery

Long essays

Short notes

1. Elevators	NTR-OR	1994 Nov	53
	NTR-OR	1999 Apr	
	NTR-NR	2004 Apr	
	NTR-NR	2005 Apr	
2. Dental elevators	NTR-OR	1997 Apr	53
	NTR-OR	1998 Oct	
3. Principles of elevators	NTR-OR	1992 Nov	53
	NTR-OR	1993 May	

Brief notes

1. Principles of elevators?	NTR-NR	2004 Oct	53

12. General Principles and Techniques of Surgery

Long essays

1. Discuss the objectives of tooth extractions.	NTR-OR	1995 Apr	
2. What are the complications of extraction of teeth? How would you avoid them? Describe in detail the treatment of any one.	NTR-OR	1982 Jun	793

Short notes

1. Principles of elevators?	NTR-OR	1992 Nov	53
2. Principles of forceps extraction?	NTR-OR	1996 Apr	53

Brief notes

13. Introduction to Exodontics

Long essays

1. Discuss in detail indications, contraindications, principles followed in dental extraction of teeth. Note on complications?	NTR-NR	2005 Oct	

Short notes

1. Complications of extraction.	NTR-OR	1995 Oct	794
	NTR-OR	1996 Oct	
	NTR-OR	2001 Apr	
	NTR-NR	2006 Oct	
2. Contraindications for extraction?	NTR-OR	1992 Nov	

Brief notes

14. Forceps Extraction

Long essays

Short notes

1. Forceps extraction	NTR-OR	1992 Apr	55

Brief notes

15. Surgical Exodontics

Long essays

Short notes

1. Transalveolar extraction	NTR-OR	1991 Oct	117
	NTR-OR	1995 Oct	
	NTR-OR	1999 Apr	
	NTR-OR	2000 Apr	
	NTR-NR	2004 Oct	
	NTR-NR	2006 Mar	
2. Open method extraction of teeth	NTR-NR	2005 Apr	117

Brief notes

16. Transplantation and Reimplantation

Long essays

Short notes

1. Tooth transplantation	NTR-OR	1994 Nov

Brief notes

1. Reimplantation?	NTR-NR	2002 Oct

17. Impacted Teeth

Long essays

1. Classify impactions and discuss the management of impactions?	NTR-OR	1991 Oct	124, 128
2. Classify the impaction of mandibular III molar tooth. How will you manage mesio-oblique impactions?	NTR-OR	1998 Oct	124, 128
3. Define impaction. Write about the classification surgical management and associated complications	NTR-OR	1993 May	124, 128
4. Classify impacted mandibular third molar. Write in detail the steps in surgical removal of impacted mandibular third molar.	NTR-NR	2006 Oct	124, 128

5. How would you extract an impacted canine from the palate surgically? Give the Pre- and post-operative management in detail.	NTR-OR	1982 Jun	130
6. What are the possible complications of an impacted lower third molar? Mentions briefly how could you access an impacted lower third molar	NTR-OR	1997 Apr	124, 124
7. What is impaction? Write the classification of impacted mandibular 3rd molar tooth. Add a note on various techniques of surgical extraction.	NTR-NR	2002 Oct	124, 134

Short notes

1. Maxillary canine impaction	NTR-OR	1999 Oct	125
2. Classification of impacted 3rd molar	NTR-OR	2000 Apr	124
3. Localization of impacted maxillary canine	NTR-OR	1996 Apr	125
4. Radiological assessment of lower third major	NTR-OR	1999 Apr	127
5. Winter's classification of impacted lower third molar	NTR-OR	2000 Apr	124
6. Clark's technique for localization of impacted maxillary	NTR-OR	2000 Apr	

Brief notes

1. Impacted tooth?	NTR-NR	2006 Apr	122
2. Define impaction of tooth?	NTR-NR	2006 Oct	122
3. List the spaces, where the lower third molar root piece can get displaced?	NTR-NR	2002 Apr	
4. Complications of impacted 3rd molar tooth?	NTR-NR	2005 Apr	134

18. Preprosthetic Surgery

Long essays

Short notes

1. Alveoloplasty	NTR-OR	1997 Apr	421
	NTR-NR	2006 Apr	
2. Alveolectomy	NTR-OR	1994 Nov	421
3. Vestibuloplasty	NTR-OR	1998 Apr	428
4. Sulcus extension?	NTR-OR	1992 Nov	
5. Pre-prosthetic surgery?	NTR-OR	1994 May	417

Brief notes

1. Dean's alveoplasty?	NTR-NR	2006 Oct	421
2. Mandibular Ridge augmentation	NTR-NR	2004 Oct	432
3. Implant supported prosthesis?	NTR-NR	2006 Apr	

19. Endodontic Surgery

Long essays

Short notes

1. Apicoectomy	NTR-OR	1998 Oct	135
	NTR-OR	2001 Oct	

Brief notes

1. Apicoectomy	NTR-NR	2005 Apr	135

20. Periodontal Surgery

Long essays

Short notes

1. Frenectomy	NTR-OR	2001 Apr	427
2. Vestibuloplasty	NTR-OR	1998 Apr	428
3. Sulcus extension	NTR-OR	1992 Nov	428

Brief notes

1. Frenectomy	NTR-NR	2002 Oct	427

21. Orthodontic Surgery

Long essays

Short notes

Brief notes

22. Orthognathic Surgery

Long essays

1. Write about facial proportions and note about class I and II prognathism and method to plan treatment by Orthognathic surgery?	NTR-NR	2006 Apr	

Short notes

1. Prognathism	NTR-OR	1997 Oct	
2. Genioplasty—Indication diagnosis technique	NTR-NR	2001 Oct	291

Brief notes

1. Treatment of mandibular prognathism	NTR-NR	2005 Apr	

23. Distraction Osteogenesis

Long essays

Short notes

Brief notes

24. Transplantation of Tissues

Long essays

Short notes

Brief notes

25. Contemporary Implant Dentistry

Long essays

Short notes

Brief notes

1. Implants?	NTR-NR	2006 Apr	

26. Surgical Considerations of Oral Neoplasms

Long essays

Short notes

Brief notes

27. Cleft Lip and Palate

Long essays

Short notes

1. Cleft lip?	NTR-OR	1994 May	547
	NTR-OR	1995 Apr	
	NTR-OR	1997 Oct	
2. Cleft palate?	NTR-OR	1991 Oct	550
	NTR-OR	1993 May	

Brief notes

1. Cleft lip and palate protocol?	NTR-NR	2005 Oct	551

28. Acquired Defects of the Hard and Soft Tissues of the Face

Long essays

Short notes

Brief notes

29. Surgical Reconstruction of Defects of the Jaws

Long essays

		Neelima		

Short notes

Brief notes

30. Maxillary Sinus Infections

Long essays

1.	Describe the clinical features and treatment of oroantral fistula	NTR-OR	1982 Jun	572
2.	What are the causes of oroantral communication Describe any one method of surgical closure of oroantral fistula?	NTR-OR	1999 Apr	572
3.	Enumerate the etiological factors of oro-antral fistula. Add a brief note on its management	NTR-OR	1998 Apr	572
4.	Describe the surgical anatomy of the maxillary sinus and merits of various surgical approaches to maxillary sinus?	NTR-OR	1991 Oct	563
5.	Discuss the surgical anatomy of maxillary sinus and write in detail the management of oroantral fistula?	NTR-NR	2006 Oct	563
6.	Define the boundaries of maxillary sinus. Describe the technique for closure of an oroantral communication encountered following extraction of maxillary first molar diagnosis postoperative care?	NTR-NR	2001 Oct	563

Short notes

1.	Maxillary sinus?	NTR-OR	1994 May	563
2.	Oro-antral fistula	NTR-OR	1996 Apr	572
3.	Antrostomy?	NTR-OR	1992 Nov	579
4.	Nasal antrostomy—indications and technique?	NTR-OR	2001 Apr	579
5.	Removal of fractured root from the maxillary sinus?	NTR-OR	1997 Oct	

Brief notes

1.	Oroantral fistula	NTR-NR	2005 Apr	572
2.	Definition of oroantral fistula and communication?	NTR-NR	2002 Apr	572

31. Space Infections

Long essays

1.	Write the clinical features, etiology and management of Ludwig's angina and note on systemic complications?	NTR-NR	2006 Apr	624

Neelima

Short notes

1. Epulis?	NTR-OR	1993 May	
2. Cancrum oris?	NTR-OR	1991 Oct	
3. Pericoronitis?	NTR-OR	1996 Apr	624
	NTR-OR	1999 Oct	
4. Periapical cyst	NTR-NR	2005 Apr	448
5. Apical granuloma?	NTR-OR	1982 Jun	
6. Acute alveolar abscess?	NTR-OR	1989 Feb	591
	NTR-OR	1994 Nov	
7. Ludwig's angina	NTR-OR	1982 Jun	624
	NTR-OR	1991 Oct	
	NTR-OR	1992 Nov	
	NTR-OR	1995 Oct	
	NTR-OR	1998 Oct	
	NTR-OR	1999 Apr	
	NTR-NR	2004 Oct	
8. Treatment of Ludwig's angina?	NTR-OR	2001 Apr	628
9. Cavernous sinus thrombosis?	NTR-OR	1982 Jun	634
10. Intratemporal space?	NTR-OR	2001 Oct	609
	NTR-NR	2002 Apr	
11. Pterygomandibular space	NTR-OR	1997 Apr	619
	NTR-OR	1999 Apr	
12. Submasseteric space infection?	NTR-OR	1998 Apr	619
13. Submandibular space infection	NTR-OR	2000 Apr	612
14. Infections of the oral cavity?	NTR-OR	1995 Apr	

Brief notes

1. Residual cyst?	NTR-NR	2006 Oct	449
2. Periapical cyst?	NTR-NR	2005 Apr	448
3. Cavernous sinus thrombosis?	NTR-NR	2005 Apr	634
4. Masticatory space infection?	NTR-NR	2006 Oct	618
5. Submandibular space boundaries?	NTR-NR	2006 Oct	612
6. Name the structures in the middle meatus?	NTR-NR	2002 Apr	632

32. Cysts of Oral Cavity

Long essays

1. How would you diagnose benign artic lesions of the jaws?	NTR-OR	1996 Apr	439
2. Classify cystic lesions of the oral cavity; discuss its pathogenesis, diagnosis and treatment?	NTR-OR	1994 May	439
3. Classify cysts. Describe the etiology, clinical features and treatment of a periapical cyst of maxillary mesisers?	NTR-NR	2001 Apr	441

4. Write etiology, clinical features, diagnosis and treatment of odontogenic keratocyst of the mandible affecting a young adult of 20 years?	NTR-NR	2002 Oct	439

Short notes

1. Keratocyst?	NTR-OR	1998 Apr	441
2. Residual cyst?	NTR-OR	1999 Apr	449
	NTR-NR	2006 Apr	
3. Radicular cyst?	NTR-OR	1999 Oct	448
4. Nasolabial cyst?	NTR-OR	1999 Apr	457
5. Periapical granuloma?	NTR-OR	1982 Jun	
6. Dentigerous cyst?	NTR-OR	1994 Nov	444
	NTR-OR	1999 Oct	
7. Traumatic bone cyst?	NTR-OR	2000 Apr	454
8. Primordial cyst?	NTR-OR	1998 Apr	441
9. Globulomaxillary cyst?	NTR-OR	2000 Apr	452
10. Benign cystic lesions of the mandible?	NTR-OR	1991 Oct	
11. Marsupialization?	NTR-OR	1998 Oct	463
	NTR-NR	2004 Oct	

Brief notes

1. Odontogenic keratocyst?	NTR-NR	2005 Oct	441
2. Difference between enucleation and marsupialization?	NTR-OR	2002 Apr	

33. Tumors of Oral Cavity

Long essays

1. Differentiate between benign and malignant tumors. Describe the signs and symptoms and management of an ameloblastoma involving the angle of the mandible?	NTR-NR	2002 Apr	481
2. How do you diagnose ameloblastoma? Outline the methods of treating this tumor involving the mandibular third molar area?	NTR-OR	1989 Feb	481

Short notes

1. Odontoma	NTR-OR	1997 Oct	491
	NTR-OR	2001 Oct	
2. Odontomes?	NTR-OR	1998 Oct	491
3. Adamantinoma?	NTR-OR	1995 Apr	481
4. Ameloblastoma?	NTR-OR	1993 May	481
	NTR-OR	1999 Apr	
5. Pindborg tumor?	NTR-OR	1999 Oct	489
6. Torus palatinus?	NTR-OR	1998 Oct	

7. Pleomorphic adenoma?	NTR-OR	1994 Nov	526
8. Adeno-ameloblastoma?	NTR-OR	1997 Oct	
9. Adenomatoid odontogenic tumor?	NTR-OR	1999 Oct	

Brief notes

34. Salivary Gland Disorders

Long essays

1. Describe the clinical features and treatment of salivary calculus of Warthin's duct.	NTR-OR	2001 Oct	519

Short notes

1. Ranula	NTR-OR	1996 Apr	524
	NTR-OR	1997 Oct	
	NTR-NR	2001 Oct	
2. Sialolith	NTR-OR	1997 Apr	519
	NTR-OR	1999 Apr	
	NTR-NR	2002 Apr	
3. Sialedenitis	NTR-OR	1993 May	
	NTR-NR	2001 Apr	520
4. Sialography	NTR-OR	1992 Nov	
	NTR-NR	2004 Apr	530
5. Pleomorphic adenoma?	NTR-OR	1994 Nov	526
6. Mixed tumor of parotid gland	NTR-NR	2005 Apr	526
7. Submandibular salivary calculi	NTR-OR	1997 Oct	519
8. Mixed tumor of parotid gland?	NTR-NR	2005 Apr	526

Brief notes

1. Ranula?	NTR-NR	2004 Apr	524
2. Mucocele?	NTR-NR	2005 Oct	523
3. Sialadenitis?	NTR-NR	2005 Oct	520
4. Adenocarcinoma of minor salivary gland in palate?	NTR-NR	2006 Apr	528

35. Facial Neuropathology/Neurological Disorders

Long essays

1. Write in detail clinical features and management of paroxysmal trigeminal neuralgia?	NTR-OR	1999 Oct	685
2. Define trigeminal neuralgia and discuss in brief its etiology, clinical signs, symptoms and management?	NTR-OR	1992 Nov	685

Short notes

1. Facial palsy?	NTR-NR	2004 Apr	719
2. Trigger zone	NTR-OR	1993 May	

			Neelima
3. Nerve injuries?	NTR-OR	1996 Apr	803
	NTR-OR	1997 Apr	
4. Trigeminal neuralgia	NTR-OR	1991 Oct	685
	NTR-OR	1994 May	
	NTR-OR	1995 Oct	
	NTR-OR	1998 Apr	
	NTR-OR	2000 Apr	
	NTR-NR	2005 Oct	
5. Treatment of trigeminal neuralgia?	NTR-OR	2001 Oct	687
6. Medical management of trigeminal neuralgia?	NTR-NR	2004 Oct	687
7. Surgical management of trigeminal neuralgia?	NTR-NR	2006 Oct	687
8. Nerve injuries following trauma in facial region?	NTR-NR	2005 Apr	
9. Analgesics for oro-facial pain?	NTR-NR	2005 Oct	

Brief notes

1. Bell's palsy?	NTR-NR	2005 Apr	719
2. Name the surgical treatment modalities for Trigeminal neuralgia?	NTR-NR	2002 Apr	689

36. Diseases of Temporomandibular Joint

Long essays

1. Describe the etiology, clinical features and management of ankylosis of T.M. joint?	NTR-OR	1997 Oct	226, 231
2. Enumerate the causes of inability to open the mouth. How would you treat a case of bony ankylosis?	NTR-OR	1999 Apr	211
3. Define ankylosis of TMJ mention the etiology. Clinical features a management of unilateral ankylosis in a 10 yrs old patient.	NTR-OR	1997 Apr	226

Short notes

1. Trismus	NTR-OR	1989 Feb	211
	NTR-OR	1994 Nov	
2. Ankylosis	NTR-OR	1993 May	226
	NTR-OR	1995 Apr	
3. Subluxation of TMJ	NTR-OR	1994 May	215
	NTR-OR	1997 Oct	
	NTR-OR	1999 Apr	
	NTR-NR	2000 Apr	
	NTR-NR	2005 Oct	
4. Temporomandibular joint?	NTR-OR	1995 Apr	205
	NTR-OR	2004 Oct	

5. Pain dysfunction of TM joint?	NTR-OR	1994 Nov	241
	NTR-OR	1996 Apr	
	NTR-OR	1999 Oct	
6. Dislocation of TM joint?	NTR-OR	1996 Apr	212
	NTR-OR	1999 Oct	
7. Acute dislocation of TM joint	NTR-OR	1998 Apr	212
8. Acute TMJ dislocation, Causes and treatment	NTR-NR	2001 Oct	212
9. Ankylosis treatment protocol	NTR-NR	2005 Apr	231
10. Surgical management of TMJ ankylosis?	NTR-NR	2006 Oct	231
11. Interposition osteoarthroplasty?	NTR-NR	2001 Apr	232

Brief notes

1. Interposition arthroplasty?	NTR-NR	2005 Oct	232
2. List the ligaments of temporomandibular joints?	NTR-NR	2002 Apr	206

37. Systemic Diseases Manifested in the Jaw Bones

Long essays

1. Describe the etiology, clinical features and the management of chronic osteomyelitis of the mandible?	NTR-OR	1997 Oct	637

Short notes

1. Osteomyelitis?	NTR-OR	1994 May	636
2. Acute osteomyelitis	NTR-NR	2002 Apr	640
3. Garre's osteomyelitis	NTR-OR	1998 Oct	656
4. Chronic suppurative osteomyelitis?	NTR-NR	2006 Oct	637
5. Chronic osteomyelitis of mandible?	NTR-NR	2006 Apr	637
6. Osteoradionecrosis?	NTR-OR	1989 Feb	662
	NTR-OR	1997 Apr	
	NTR-OR	1998 Apr	
7. Hyperbaric oxygen therapy?	NTR-NR	2001 Apr	646

Brief notes

1. Hyperbaric oxygen therapy?	NTR-NR	2002 Oct	646
	NTR-NR	2004 Oct	
2. Hyperbaric oxygen therapy indications?	NTR-NR	2002 Apr	646
3. Classification of osteomyelitis of jaw bones?	NTR-NR	2004 Oct	639

38. Premalignant Lesion, Premalignant Conditions and Oral Cancer

Long essays

Short notes

1. Leukoplakia?	NTR-OR	1997 Oct	727
2. Submucous fibrosis?	NTR-OR	1997 Oct	729

				Neelima
3.	Analgesics in OMF surgery?	NTR-NR	2002 Oct	149
4.	Squamous cell carcinoma of lip?	NTR-NR	2004 Apr	
5.	Premalignant conditions?	NTR-NR	2006 Apr	729

Brief notes

1.	Radiotherapy?	NTR-NR	2002 Oct	732
2.	Staging of tumor?	NTR-NR	2005 Oct	732
3.	Radiotherapy for oral carcinoma?	NTR-NR	2006 Apr	732

39. Introduction, Etiology and Changing Patterns of Maxillofacial Trauma

Long essays

1.	Describe various fractures of Jaws	NTR-OR	1994 Nov	327
2.	Write the golden hour of trauma importance and note on protocol to be followed in road traffic accident victim management and on life support system?	NTR-NR	2005 Apr	316

Short notes

1.	Tuberosity fracture?	NTR-OR	1994 May	
2.	Pathological fractures?	NTR-OR	1998 Oct	
3.	Emergency radiology in facial injury?	NTR-OR	1995 Apr	

Brief notes

40. Traumatic Injuries of Teeth and Alveolar Process

Long essays

Short notes

1.	Fractured root at middle 1/3rd?			
2.	Management of dentoalveolar fracture?	NTR-NR	2006 Oct	

Brief notes

41. Fractures of Middle Third of Face and Its Management

Long essays

1.	Describe the lines of LeFort I and II fractures. Describe the clinical features and treatment of LeFort I fractures?	NTR-OR	2001 Apr	354
2.	Write the clinical features and treatment of LeFort III fractures of midface?	NTR-NR	2005 Oct	356

Neelima

3. Define fracture. Classify the fracture of middle third of facial skeleton and write in brief the clinical signs, symptoms, diagnosis, management of Gueirns fracture?	NTR-OR	1992 Nov	353

Short notes

1. LeFort I fracture	NTR-OR	1997 Oct	354
2. LeFort II fracture	NTR-NR	2002 Apr	355
3. Diplopia	NTR-OR	1996 Apr	360
	NTR-OR	1998 Apr	
4. CSF rhinorrhea	NTR-OR	1997 Apr	357

Brief notes

42. Fractures of Zygomatic Bone and Its Management

Long essays

1. Describe the fractures of zygomatic complex and their management.	NTR-OR	1995 Apr	358, 369
2. Describe classification and clinical features of zygomatic bone complex. Write the indications for surgical treatment.	NTR-OR	1999 Oct	358, 369
3. Classify fractures of zygomatico-complex and write about the clinical features and management of fractures of zygomatic arch?	NTR-NR	2004 Oct	358, 369
4. Describe the clinical findings of zygomatic complex fracture. Enumerate the various methods of reducing the zygomatic arch fracture and discuss any one in detail?	NTR-NR	2002 Apr	358, 369

Short notes

1. Zygomatic fractures.	NTR-OR	1998 Oct	
2. Blow out fracture of orbit?	NTR-NR	2006 Apr	

Brief notes

43. Mandibular Fractures and Its Management

Long essays

1. Classify fractures of maxilla and mandible. Discuss the management of mandibular fractures.	NTR-OR	1993 May	380
2. Classify fractures of maxilla and mandible. How would you treat a case of fracture mandible in angle region?	NTR-OR	1999 Apr	380

Neelima

3. Describer the management of a case of fracture of angle of mandible, distal to the III molar tooth.	NTR-OR	1998 Oct	386

Short notes

1. Gunning splint	NTR-NR	2005 Oct	335
2. Transosseous wiring?	NTR-OR	1999 Oct	339
3. Rigid internal fixation?	NTR-NR	2002 Oct	329
4. Fracture of body of mandible?	NTR-OR	1994 Nov	
5. Dental wiring (write osteosynthesis)?	NTR-NR	2004 Apr	
6. Fracture of body of mandible in children?	NTR-OR	1998 Apr	386
7. Fracture of the body of edentulous mandible?	NTR-OR	1997 Oct	

Brief notes

1. Eyelet wiring?	NTR-NR	2004 Oct	332
2. Classification of mandibular condylar fractures?	NTR-NR	2004 Oct	403

44. Fractures of Condylar Process and Its Management

Long essays

1. Classify fracture of condyle. How would you treat a case of law subcondylar fracture	NTR-OR	2000 Apr	403, 406
2. Describe the signs, symptoms, diagnosis and treatment of bilateral condylar fractures.	NTR-OR	1982 Jun	406, 407

Short notes

1. Condylar fracture in children	NTR-OR	1998 Oct	403
2. Condylar fracture of mandible	NTR-NR	2005 Apr	403
3. How do you manage a case of unilateral condylar fracture with displacement in adults?	NTR-OR	1989 Feb	409

Brief notes

1. Treatment options for submandibular fractures?	NTR-NR	2002 Oct	409

45. Healing of Fracture and Wounds

Long essays

Short notes

1. Healing of extraction wound?	NTR-NR	2004 Apr

Brief notes

1. Malunion	NTR-NR	2002 Oct
2. Healing of extraction wound?	NTR-NR	2006 Apr

Neelima

46. Emergencies in Dental Practice

Long essays

Short notes

Brief notes

1. Significance of AIDS in dentistry?	NTR-NR	2006 Oct	780
2. Prophylactic antibiotics regimen for cardiac compromised patient?	NTR-NR	2002 Oct	115

47. Complications in Oral Surgery

Long essays

Short notes

1. Syncope	NTR-OR	1994 Apr	
	NTR-OR	1998 Oct	
	NTR-OR	1999 Apr	
2. Dry socket	NTR-OR	1996 Apr	802
	NTR-OR	1999 Apr	
	NTR-NR	2006 Oct	
3. Anaphylaxis?	NTR-OR	2001 Apr	

Brief notes

1. Syncope?	NTR-NR	2006 Oct	
2. Dry socket?	NTR-NR	2002 Oct	802
3. Anaphylaxis?	NTR-NR	2004 Apr	
	NTR-NR	2005 Apr	

48. Hemorrhage and Shock

Long essays

Short notes

1. Hemophilia?	NTR-OR	1998 Apr	769
2. Hemorrhagic shock?	NTR-NR	2006 Oct	
3. Shock in oral surgery?	NTR-OR	1995 Apr	
	NTR-OR	1998 Apr	
4. Blood groups?	NTR-OR	1992 Nov	
5. Blood grouping and transfusion?	NTR-OR	1994 Nov	
6. Autologous blood transfusion?	NTR-NR	2004 Oct	
7. Blood transfusion reactions?	NTR-NR	2002 Apr	
	NTR-NR	2006 Oct	
8. Postextraction bleeding?	NTR-OR	1993 May	
	NTR-OR	1994 Nov	

9. Management of hemorrhage in oral surgery?	NTR-NR	2002 Apr	762
10. Postextractions hemorrhage management?	NTR-NR	2005 Apr	
11. Management of post extraction hemorrhage?	NTR-NR	2004 Oct	
12. Hemophilia patient for dental extraction?	NTR-NR	2006 Apr	769

Brief notes

49. Oral and Maxillofacial Surgical Considerations in Pediatric and Geriatric Patients

Long essays

Short notes

1. Condylar fractures in children?	NTR-OR	1998 Oct	403
2. Fracture of body of the mandible in children?	NTR-OR	1998 Apr	

Brief notes

50. Miscellaneous Topics

Long essays

Short notes

1. Tracheostomy?	NTR-NR	2001 Oct	51
2. Cryosurgery?	NTR-OR	1994 May	57
	NTR-OR	1995 Apr	
	NTR-OR	1998 Oct	
3. Cryosurgery—Principles and indications in oral lesions?	NTR-OR	2001 Apr	57
4. Carotid ligation?	NTR-OR	1992 Nov	
5. Open cap splint osteosynthesis?	NTR-NR	2006 Apr	
6. Preanesthetic preparation of a patient?	NTR-OR	2001 Apr	147
7. Champy's osteosynthesis line for monocortical plating?	NTR-NR	2006 Apr	347

Brief notes

1. Pathways of pain?	NTR-NR	2006 Oct	683
2. Apert's syndrome?	NTR-NR	2006 Apr	
3. Risdon's incision?	NTR-NR	2004 Apr	
4. Giant cell lesions?	NTR-NR	2004 Apr	
5. Incision Intraorally?	NTR-NR	2004 Apr	
6. Incision and drainage?	NTR-NR	2002 Oct	
7. Functional neck dissection?	NTR-NR	2005 Apr	
8. Intraligamentary anesthesia?	NTR-NR	2006 Oct	

LOCAL ANESTHESIA

SYLLABUS

Introduction

- Neurology of facial pain
- Historical aspects, definition, types of LA, indications and contraindication, advantage and disadvantage.
- Local anesthetic drugs, classification.
- Ideal requirements of LA solutions, composition and mode of action.
- Factors to be considered in the choice of particular mode of anesthesia.
- Complications of LA, its prevention and management.

Anesthesia of Mandible

- Anatomical consideration, infiltration, mental nerve block and Inferior dental nerve block.

Anesthesia of Maxilla

- Anatomical considerations, infiltration, infraorbital block, posterior superior alveolar and maxillary nerve block.
- Extraoral blocks—Indications and technique.

General Anesthesia

- History of GA
- Indications of GA, in oral surgery
- Preanesthetic evaluation of the patient
- Premedication
- Types of GA, including IV sedation
- Stages of GA, common general anesthetic agents
- Complications during and after anesthesia
- Postanesthetic care of the patients.

SCHEME OF EXAMINATION

Theory

Theory – 70 Marks
Viva Voce – 10 Marks
Internal Assessment (Theory) – 20 Marks

Local Anesthesia (Part-A + Part-B / 35 + 35 = 70)

Subject	*Type of question*	*Marks offered*	*Total*
Part-A/Local Anesthesia	Long essays	9	1 x 9 = 09
	Short notes	4	4 x 4 = 16
	Brief notes	2	5 x 2 = 10
Part-B/Local Anesthesia	Long essays	9	1 x 9 = 09
	Short notes	4	4 x 4 = 16
	Brief notes	2	5 x 2 = 10

Clinicals

Clinicals – 70 Marks
Viva Voce – 10 Marks
Internal Assessment (Clinicals) – 20 Marks

REFERENCE BOOK

Local Anesthesia: Textbook of Local Anesthesia – By Stanely F Malamed

AUTHOR ABBREVIATION

Malamed: Stanely F Malamed

Edition: 6th

QUESTION BANK ABBREVIATION

Question Bank

LE — Long essays
SN — Short notes
BN — Brief notes

University

NTRUHS — Nandamuri Taraka Rama Rao University of Health Sciences
NTRUHS-NR — NTRUHS–New Regulations
NTRUHS-OR — NTRUHS–Old Regulations

CONTENTS

LOCAL ANESTHESIA

Malamed

1. Pain

Long essays

Short notes

Brief notes

2. Trigeminal Nerve

Long essays

1. Enumerate in detail the course of mandibular branch of trigeminal nerve and explain the technique of classical pterygomandibular nerve block?	NTR-NR	2004 Oct	188, 228

Short notes

Brief notes

3. Regional Analgesia

Long essays

Short notes

1. Nerve block?	NTR-OR	1995 Apr	188

Brief notes

4. Techniques of Regional Anesthesia and Analgesia

Long essays

1. Define the boundaries of Pterygomandibular fossa. Describe any one technique of blocking the inferior dental nerve?	NTR-OR	1982 Jun	228
2. Describe the technique of inferior dental nerve block anesthesia. Enumerate the complications of the technique?	NTR-OR	1998 Apr	228
3. Discuss in detail about surgical anatomy, indications and contraindications and technique of inferior alveolar nerve block anesthesia?	NTR-NR	2004 Apr	228

			Malamed
4. Enumerate in detail the course of mandibular branch of trigeminal nerve and explain the technique of classical pterygomandibular nerve block?	NTR-NR	2004 Oct	198

Short notes

1. Complications of inferior alveolar nerve block?	NTR-NR	2000 Apr	202
2. Inferior alveolar nerve block action of it?	NTR-NR	2006 Apr	201
3. Posterior superior alveolar nerve block anesthesia?	NTR-NR	2005 Oct	192

Brief notes

1. Give the order of anaesthetizing various nerves in direct pterygomandibular block technique?	NTR-NR	2002 Apr	228

5. Local Anesthetics and Anesthetic Solutions

Long essays

1. Discuss the indications and contraindications of local anesthesia?	NTR-OR	1994 Nov	
2. Define local anesthesia. What are the components of a standard local anesthetic solution? Discuss the indications and contraindications of local anesthesia?	NTR-OR	1994 May	03
3. Discuss about pharmacology, composition and indications for use of local anaesthetic agent. Write a note on complications of inferior alveolar anesthesia?	NTR-NR	2005 Mar	27

Short notes

1. Lignocaine hydrochloride?	NTR-NR	2002 Oct	146
2. Ideal local anesthetic drug?	NTR-OR	1991 Oct	146
3. Local anaesthetic solution?	NTR-OR	1992 Nov	27
4. Local anaesthetic agent pharmacology?	NTR-NR	2006 Apr	27
5. Contents of local anaesthetic solutions?	NTR-OR	1996 Apr	320
6. Composition of local anaesthetic solution?	NTR-NR	2004 Oct	
7. Properties of an ideal local anesthetic drug?	NTR-NR	2001 Apr	

Brief notes

1. Composition of local anesthetic solution	NTR-NR	2002 Oct	

6. Vasoconstrictors

Long essays

Short notes

			Malamed

Brief notes

1. Vasoconstrictor?	NTR-NR	2002 Oct	41
2. Role of vasoconstrictor in local anaesthetic solution?	NTR-NR	2002 Apr	41

7. Preanesthetic Evaluation Choice of Anesthetics

Long essays

Short notes

Brief notes

8. Anesthetic Complications and Office Emergencies

Long essays

Short notes

Brief notes

9. Conscious Sedation in Dentistry

Long essays

Short notes

Brief notes

10. Postoperative Pain Control

Long essays

Short notes

Brief notes

11. Armamentarium

Long essays

Short notes

Brief notes

12. Sterilization

Long essays

Malamed

Short notes

Brief notes

13. Dentistry, Local Anesthesia and the Law

Long essays

Short notes

Brief notes

14. Miscellaneous Topics

Long essays

Short notes

1. General anesthetic drugs?	NTR-OR	Apr 1995
2. Stages of general anesthesia?	NTR-OR	May 1993
3. Indications for general anesthesia?	NTR-NR	Apr 2004
4. General anesthesia vs local anesthesia?	NTR-NR	Oct 2005

Brief notes

1. Gaseous anesthetic agent?	NTR-NR	Apr 2006

PERIODONTICS

SYLLABUS

1. Introduction, scope and applicability of the subject, historical background of periodontology
2. Maintenance of health – role and scope of the oral physiotherapy measures, patient education programmes and periodic check-ups
3. Classification of gingival and periodontal diseases
4. Gingival enlargements
5. Infective muco-gingival conditions – specific and non-specific
6. Degenerative conditions – Desquamative lesions
7. Atrophic conditions affecting gingival and periodontal tissues
8. Local and systemic factors in the causation of the gingival and periodontal lesions
9. Periodontitis and squela
10. Basic considerations in occlusal rehabilitations
11. Diagnosis and diagnostic aids including roentgenographic and its uses and limitations
12. Prognosis
13. Morphological defects of the muco-gingival structures influencing periodontium and their treatment
14. Treatment of all gingival and periodontal disturbances – treatment planning phases, rationale, different available therapeutic procedures and healing mechanism
15. Role of nutrition in etiology and treatment
16. Drugs in periodontics
17. Instrumentation
18. Splints
19. Preventive periodontics, concepts of focal infections
20. Materials used in periodontia
21. Epidemiology of periodontal disease with special emphasis to India
22. Epidemiological indices
23. Special emphasis on medically compromised patients
24. Basic concepts of implants

SCHEME OF EXAMINATION

Theory

Theory – 70 Marks
Viva Voce – 10 Marks
Internal Assessment (Theory) – 20 Marks

Periodontics (Part-A + Part-B / 35 + 35 = 70)

Subject	*Type of question*	*Marks offered*	*Total*
Part-A/Periodontics	Long essays	9	1 x 9 = 09
	Short notes	4	4 x 4 = 16
	Brief notes	2	5 x 2 = 10
Part-B/Periodontics	Long essays	9	1 x 9 = 09
	Short notes	4	4 x 4 = 16
	Brief notes	2	5 x 2 = 10

Clinicals

Clinicals – 70 Marks
Viva Voce – 10 Marks
Internal Assessment (Clinicals) – 20 Marks

REFERENCE BOOK

Periodontics: Essentials of Clinical Periodontics and Periodontology – By Shanti Priya Reddy

AUTHOR ABBREVIATION

Shanti: Shanti Priya Reddy

Edition: 2nd

QUESTION BANK ABBREVIATION

Question Bank

LE — Long essays
SN — Short notes
BN — Brief notes

University

NTRUHS — Nandamuri Taraka Rama Rao University of Health Sciences
NTRUHS-NR — NTRUHS–New Regulations
NTRUHS-OR — NTRUHS–Old Regulations

CONTENTS

Contd...

Contd...

Contd...

Contd...

Contd...

Contd...

PERIODONTICS

Shanti

1. The Historical Background of Periodontology

Long essays

Short notes

Brief notes

2. Introduction to Evidence-based Decision Making

Long essays

Short notes

Brief notes

3. Assessing Evidence

Long essays

Short notes

Brief notes

4. Implementing Evidence-based Decision in Clinical Practice

Long essays

Short notes

Brief notes

5. The Gingiva

Long essays

1. Describe briefly the importance of attached gingiva	NTR-NR	1990 Jul	9
2. Define Gingiva. Describe its macroscopic and microscopic appearance and functions. Add a note on importance of gingival fluid.	NTR-OR	1998 Apr	9
3. Write about histological and functional features of normal gingiva. Add a note on role of epithelial attachment in periodontal disease.	NTR-NR	1999 Oct	8

Shanti

Short notes

1. Gingival fibers	NTR-NR	1989 Jul	8, 15
2. Attached gingiva	NTR-NR	1994 May	8, 9
	NTR-NR	2004 May	
3. Sulcular epithelium	NTR-NR	2001 Apr	12
4. Enzymes in gingiva	NTR-NR	1997 Oct	137
5. Junctional epithelium	NTR-NR	1988 Jan	12
	NTR-OR	1994 Nov	
	NTR-OR	1995 Oct	
	NTR-NR	2002 Oct	
6. Dentogingival junction	NTR-NR	2004 Oct	13
7. Gingival pigmentation	NTR-OR	1993 May	

Brief notes

1. Gingival col	NTR-NR	2005 Mar	9
2. Free gingiva	NTR-NR	2006 Oct	8
3. Long Junctional epithelium	NTR-NR	2005 Mar	12

6. The Tooth-Supporting Structures

Long essays

1. Describe the structure and functions of periodontic ligament	NTR-NR	1988 Jan	16, 20
2. Describe briefly the various gingival and periodontal fiber groups	NTR-NR	1990 Jul	15, 18
3. Describe in detail the role of alveolar bone in health and periodontal disease	NTR-NR	1997 Apr	22
4. Define periodontal ligament. Describe its microscopic features. Add a note on its functions	NTR-NR	2002 Oct	16, 20
5. Define periodontal ligament. Describe the microscopic and macroscopic features of periodontal ligament	NTR-NR	1995 Apr	16
6. Define Cementum. Describe structure composition, and clinical significance of cementum?	NTR-OR	1994 May	25, 26
7. Enumerate the principle groups of periodontal ligament fibers. Add a note on its cellular elements and functions of periodontal ligament?	NTR-NR	2005 Oct	18, 20

Short notes

1. Dehiscence	NTR-NR	1997 Apr	23
2. Fenestration	NTR-NR	2000 Apr	23
3. Lamina dura	NTR-OR	1994 May	22
	NTR-NR	2004 Oct	
	NTR-NR	2006 Apr	
4. Oxytalin fibers	NTR-NR	1995 Apr	17, 19

5. A cellular cementum	NTR-NR	2004 Oct	25
6. Cellular cementum?	NTR-NR	2001 Oct	25
7. Intermediate plexus?	NTR-OR	1994 Nov	
8. Mediator of alveolar bone	NTR-NR	1990 Jul	24
9. Composition of cementum	NTR-NR	2002 Apr	25
	NTR-NR	2004 Oct	
10. Cementoenamel junction	NTR-NR	1994 May	26
	NTR-NR	2004 May	
	NTR-NR	2005 Mar	
11. Fenestration and dehiscence	NTR-NR	1988 Jul	23
	NTR-OR	1994 Nov	
	NTR-OR	1995 Oct	
	NTR-NR	2002 Oct	
12. Dehiscence and fenestration?	NTR-OR	1983 July	23
13. Cementoenamel junction relationships	NTR-NR	1998 Apr	26
14. Physical functions of periodontal ligament	NTR-NR	2000 Apr	20

Brief notes

7. Aging and the Periodontium

Long essays

Short notes

Brief notes

1. Age changes in the periodontium?	NTR-NR	2003 Apr	30

8. Classification of Diseases and Conditions Affecting the Periodontium

Long essays

Short notes

Brief notes

9. Epidemiology of Gingival and Periodontal Diseases

Long essays

1. Define dental epidemiology and write in detail about the indices used in assessing gingival inflammation	NTR-OR	2001 Apr	41
2. "Periodontal health for all by 2000 AD" what do you understand by this statement. How are you going to implement it by systematic manner?	NTR-OR	1997 Oct	

Short notes

1. CPITN	NTR-NR	1995 Apr	
	NTR-OR	1997 Oct	
2. Russell's index	NTR-NR	1997 Apr	46
3. Sillines and loe index	NTR-NR	1993 May	49
4. Bleeding Point index	NTR-OR	1994 May	45
5. Oral hygiene simplified	NTR-NR	1989 Jun	48
6. Russell's periodontal index	NTR-NR	1989 Jul	46
7. Periodontal disease index	NTR-NR	2001 Apr	46
8. Ideal requirements of an index	NTR-NR	2002 Apr	43

Brief notes

10. Microbiology of Periodontal Diseases

Long essays

1. Describe the role of microorganisms in the etiology of periodontal diseases?	NTR-OR	1996 Apr	60
2. Define and classify dental plaque? Write in detail about its composition and ill effects?	NTR-NR	2003 Apr	57
3. Define and classify microbial plaque. Discuss the role of microbial plaque in the etiology of gingival and periodontal disease?	NTR-NR	2005 Oct	57

Short notes

1. Materia alba	NTR-NR	2000 Apr	452
2. Acquired pellicle?	NTR-NR	2002 Oct	456
3. Subgingival plaque	NTR-NR	1993 May	58
	NTR-OR	1998 Apr	
4. Specific plaque hypothesis?	NTR-NR	2006 Oct	62
5. Differences between supra and subgingival plaque	NTR-NR	1991 Oct	58

Brief notes

1. Specific plaque hypothesis?	NTR-NR	2002 Oct	62

11. Role of Dental Calculus and Other Predisposing Factors

Long essays

Short notes

1. Calculus	NTR-NR	1992 Nov	66
2. Food impaction	NTR-OR	1996 Apr	71
	NTR-OR	1998 Oct	
	NTR-OR	1999 Oct	

			Shanti
3. Subgingival calculus	NTR-NR	2001 Apr	66
4. Attachment of calculus	NTR-NR	1998 Oct	68
	NTR-NR	2000 Apr	
5. Theories of calculus formation	NTR-NR	1983 Jul	68
	NTR-OR	1990 Jul	
	NTR-OR	1997 Apr	
	NTR-NR	2002 Oct	
6. Difference between supra- and subgingival calculus?	NTR-OR	1997 Oct	68

Brief notes

1. Food impaction	NTR-NR	2004 Apr	71
	NTR-NR	2006 Oct	

12. Genetic Factors Associated with Periodontal Diseases

Long essays

Short notes

Brief notes

13. Immunity and Inflammation—Basic Concepts

Long essays

Short notes

1. IgG?	NTR-OR	2001 Oct	
2. Mast cell	NTR-NR	1999 Oct	17
	NTR-NR	2002 Apr	
3. Lymphocyte	NTR-NR	1999 Apr	81
4. Immunoglobulins	NTR-NR	2006 Oct	84, 113
5. Arthus reaction	NTR-NR	1999 Oct	

Brief notes

1. Cytokines	NTR-NR	2005 Oct	110
2. Neutrophils	NTR-NR	2006 Apr	78
3. Name the functional defects of leukocytes	NTR-NR	2000 Apr	

14. Microbial Interactions with the Host in Periodontal Diseases

Long essays

Short notes

Brief notes

15. Smoking and Periodontal Diseases

Long essays

Short notes

Brief notes

16. Molecular Biology of the Host-Microbe Interactions in Periodontal Diseases

Long essays

Short notes

Brief notes

17. Host Modulations

Long essays

Short notes

Brief notes

18. Influence of Systemic Disorders and Stress on the Periodontium

Long essays

Short notes

1. Vitamin C	NTR-NR	2001 Apr	96
2. Chediak-Higashi syndrome	NTR-OR	1994 May	99
3. Diabetes and periodontal health	NTR-NR	2005 Apr	100
4. Oral lesions in diabetes mellitus	NTR-NR	1997 Apr	
5. Diabetes mellitus and periodontal disease	NTR-NR	2000 Apr	100
6. Periodontal manifestations of diabetes mellitus?	NTR-NR	2006 Apr	100

Brief notes

19. Periodontal Medicine: Impact of Periodontal Infection on Systemic Health

Long essays

Short notes

1. Tuberculous sclerosis?	NTR-OR	1994 May	

Brief notes

20. Oral Malodor

Long essays

Shanti

Short notes

1. Halitosis	NTR-NR	1989 Jan	106
	NTR-OR	1992 Nov	
	NTR-OR	1997 Apr	
	NTR-OR	1998 Apr	
	NTR-NR	2001 Apr	
	NTR-NR	2003 Apr	

Brief notes

21. Defense Mechanisms of Gingiva

Long essays

1. Describe the defense mechanism of gingiva	NTR-NR	1994 Nov	131

Short notes

1. Gingival fluid	NTR-NR	1988 Jan	131
	NTR-OR	1992 Nov	
	NTR-OR	1995 Apr	
2. Enzymes in gingiva?	NTR-OR	1997 Oct	137
3. Gingival crevicular fluid?	NTR-OR	2001 Oct	131
4. Disease activity and inactivity?	NTR-NR	2002 Apr	
5. Composition of gingival cervical fluid?	NTR-NR	2003 Apr	135
6. Methods of collection of Gingival crevicular fluid (GCF)	NTR-NR	2005 Oct	134

Brief notes

22. Gingival Inflammation

Long essays

Short notes

1. Enumerate the stages of gingivitis	NTR-NR	1995 Oct	140
2. Pathways of gingival inflammation	NTR-NR	1998 Oct	
3. Established lesion of chronic gingivitis	NTR-NR	1990 Jul	141

Brief notes

23. Clinical Features of Gingivitis

Long essays

1. Discuss gingival bleeding?	NTR-OR	1983 July	144
2. Define gingival bleeding. Write about causes and management of gingival bleeding	NTR-NR	2001 Apr	144

3. Define and classify gingival recession. Discuss in detail the etiology, and management of gingival recession?	NTR-NR	2004 Apr	148

Short notes

1. Gingival recession	NTR-NR	1998 Oct	148
	NTR-NR	2001 Oct	
2. Gingival pigmentations	NTR-OR	1993 May	
3. Management of operative bleeding	NTR-NR	2000 Apr	
4. Management of localized gingival bleeding	NTR-NR	1997 Oct	

Brief notes

1. Stillman's clefts?	NTR-NR	2001 Apr	419
	NTR-NR	2006 Apr	
2. Etiology of gingival recession	NTR-NR	2002 Oct	148
3. Classify the gingival recession?	NTR-NR	2003 Apr	148
4. Enumerate the stages of gingivitis?	NTR-NR	2002 Apr	140

24. Gingival Enlargements

Long essays

1. Classify gingival enlargement and write in detail about phenytoin enlargement	NTR-NR	1989 Jul	151
2. Classify gingival enlargement and describe the drug induced gingival enlargements.	NTR-NR	2006 Oct	151
3. Classify gingival enlargement. Discuss the histopathology and clinical features of drug induced gingival enlargement (DIGO)	NTR-NR	2005 Apr	151
4. Define gingival enlargement. Write briefly the differential diagnosis of inflammatory non-Inflammatory gingival enlargement	NTR-NR	1990 Jul	151

Short notes

1. Angiogranuloma	NTR-NR	2005 Mar	160
2. Pregnancy gingivitis	NTR-NR	2000 Apr	159
	NTR-NR	2001 Apr	
	NTR-NR	2006 Apr	
3. Benign tumors of gingiva	NTR-NR	1995 Oct	164
4. Leukemic gingival enlargement	NTR-NR	1996 Apr	161
	NTR-OR	1999 Oct	
5. Conditioned gingival enlargement	NTR-NR	1996 Apr	159
6. Drug induced gingival enlargements	NTR-NR	1993 May	154
	NTR-OR	1997 Oct	

Brief notes

25. Acute Gingival Infections

Long essays

1.	Discuss the clinical features, histopathology and management of gingivosis	NTR-NR	1989 Jul	172
2.	Describe the etiology, clinical features and treatment of acute necrotizing ulcerative gingivitis	NTR-NR	1998 Oct	168
3.	Describe the etiology, clinical features and differential diagnosis of acute herpetic gingiva stomatitis	NTR-NR	2000 Apr	171
4.	Enumerate the acute infections of gingiva describe the etiology. Clinical features. And histopathology of acute necrotizing ulcerative gingivitis	NTR-NR	2002 Apr	167
5.	Enumerate the acute lesions of gingiva and write in detail the clinical features. Histopathology and management of acute necrotizing ulcerative gingivitis	NTR-NR	1989 Jan	167

Short notes

1.	Pericoronitis	NTR-NR	1997 Oct	175
		NTR-OR	1999 Apr	
2.	Aphthous ulcer	NTR-NR	1998 Apr	173
3.	Gingival abscess?	NTR-OR	1997 Apr	152
4.	Hepatic gingivostomatitis	NTR-OR	1999 Apr	172
		NTR-NR	2006 Apr	
5.	Acute hepatic gingivostomatitis?	NTR-NR	2001 Oct	172
6.	Treatment of ANUG?	NTR-OR	1997 Oct	170

Brief notes

1.	Porphyromonas gingivalis?	NTR-NR	2005 Oct	244

26. Gingival Diseases in Childhood

Long essays

Short notes

Brief notes

27. Desquamative Gingivitis

Long essays

1.	Classify Desquamative gingivitis lesions and describe in detail the candidiasis lesions?	NTR-NR	2004 May	185

Short notes

1.	Desquamative gingivitis	NTR-NR	1995 Oct	185
		NTR-OR	1998 Oct	

				Shanti
2. Herpetic gingivostomatitis?	NTR-OR	1999 Apr	172	
3. Define and classify chronic desquamative gingivitis lesions?	NTR-NR	2003 Apr	185	

Brief notes

28. Periodontal Pocket

Long essays

1. Define and classify periodontal pockets. Add a note on its histopathology and management	NTR-OR	1989 Jul	192
2. Define periodontal pocket. Describe its classification, histopathology, pathogenesis and sequale?	NTR-OR	1997 Oct	192
3. Define periodontal pocket, classify periodontal pocket. Discuss the pathogenesis and contents of periodontal pocket	NTR-NR	1998 Oct	192
4. Define periodontal pocket. Describe the non-surgical treatment regimen, which will help in pocket elimination	NTR-OR	1988 Jan	192
5. Classify periodontal pockets. Describe the clinical and microscopic features of the pocket?	NTR-NR	2006 Apr	192

Short notes

1. Suprabony pockets	NTR-NR	1992 May	200
	NTR-OR	1994 Apr	
2. Infrabony pocket	NTR-OR	1993 May	200
	NTR-OR	1996 Apr	
3. Classification of periodontal pockets	NTR-NR	2004 Oct	192
4. Root surface changes in periodontal pocket	NTR-NR	2002 Oct	198

Brief notes

29. Bone Loss and Patterns of Bone Destruction

Long essays

Short notes

1. Lipping?	NTR-OR	2001 Oct	89
2. Osseous defects	NTR-NR	1993 May	205
	NTR-OR	1995 Oct	
	NTR-NR	2006 Apr	206
3. Intrabony defects	NTR-NR	1999 Apr	208
4. Osseous deformity	NTR-NR	1983 Jul	
	NTR-OR	1988 Jul	
5. Angular bone defects	NTR-NR	1999 Apr	205
	NTR-OR	1999 Oct	

				Shanti
6. Positive architecture of alveolar bone?	NTR-NR	2001 Oct	331	
7. Mediators of alveolar bone destruction?	NTR-OR	1990 Jul	204	

Brief notes

1. Reverse architecture?	NTR-NR	2005 Oct	331
2. Inconsistent bony margins?	NTR-NR	2006 Oct	
3. Enumerate bone destructive patterns in periodontal diseases?	NTR-NR	2002 Oct	205

30. Periodontal Response to External Forces

Long essays

1. Define "Trauma from occlusion" and discuss its etiology, clinical features and management.	NTR-NR	1989 Jan	87
2. Define trauma from occlusion. Discuss the pathology, clinical and radiographic features of trauma from occlusion?	NTR-NR	2001 Oct	87
3. Describe the role of trauma from occlusion in case of periodontal diseases. Describe the physiological and pathological tooth mobility seen in the teeth involved in trauma from occlusion?	NTR-OR	1988 Jan	87

Short notes

1. Forces of occlusion?	NTR-NR	2004 May	
2. Pathology migration?	NTR-NR	2004 May	92
3. Pathological tooth migration?	NTR-OR	1993 May	92
4. Define and classify trauma from occlusion	NTR-NR	2004 Apr	87
5. Classification and diagnosis of trauma from occlusion	NTR-NR	2005 Mar	87

Brief notes

31. Masticatory System Disorders

Long essays

Short notes

1. Bruxism	NTR-NR	1989 Jan	74
	NTR-OR	1994 May	
	NTR-OR	1997 Apr	
	NTR-OR	1998 Oct	
	NTR-OR	1999 Oct	74
2. Night guard	NTR-NR	1999 Apr	
3. Masticatory cycle?	NTR-NR	2004 May	

Shanti

Brief notes

1. Facets?	NTR-NR	2000 Apr	

32. Chronic Periodontitis

Long essays

Short notes

Brief notes

33. Necrotizing Ulcerative Periodontitis, Refractory Periodontitis and Periodontitis as a Manifestation of Systemic Diseases

Long essays

Short notes

1. Refractory periodontitis	NTR-NR	1993 May	219
	NTR-OR	1996 Apr	
	NTR-OR	2004 Apr	
	NTR-NR	2002 Oct	
2. Necrotizing ulcerative periodontitis	NTR-NR	1994 Nov	218

Brief notes

1. Necrotizing ulcerative periodontitis (NUP)?	NTR-NR	2005 Oct	218

34. Aggressive Periodontitis

Long essays

1. Describe the signs, symptoms, etiology and treatment of localized juvenile periodontitis	NTR-NR	1995 Oct	214
2. Describe the signs, symptoms, differential diagnosis and treatment of localized juvenile periodontitis	NTR-OR	1993 Oct	214
3. Describe in detail about the juvenile periodontitis. Enumerate the differences between the juvenile periodontitis and adult periodontitis?	NTR-OR	1983 Jul	214

Short notes

1. Pre-pubertal periodontitis?	NTR-OR	1994 Nov	
2. Localized juvenile periodontitis	NTR-NR	2000 Apr	213
	NTR-NR	2006 Oct	
3. Localized aggressive periodontitis	NTR-NR	2005 Mar	213
4. Microorganisms in juvenile periodontitis	NTR-NR	1998 Apr	213
5. Clinical and radiographic features of localized juvenile periodontitis	NTR-NR	2002 Oct	214

Brief notes

1. P. gingivalis?	NTR-NR	2006 Oct	111
2. Actinobacillus actinomycetemeomitans?	NTR-NR	2004 Oct	215

35. Pathology and Management of Periodontal Problems in Patients with HIV Infections

Long essays

Short notes

1. Tests for AIDS	NTR-OR	1998 Oct	223
2. HIV periodontitis	NTR-OR	1999 Oct	223
3. HIV associated periodontitis	NTR-OR	1999 Apr	223
4. Periodontal manifestations of HIV infection?	NTR-NR	2006 Oct	223
5. Oral manifestations of HIV infections?	NTR-NR	2002 Oct	225

Brief notes

1. ELISA?	NTR-NR	2000 Apr	253

36. Clinical Diagnosis

Long essays

1. Describe the diagnostic aids used in periodontal diseases?	NTR-NR	2001 Oct

Short notes

1. Tooth mobility	NTR-NR	1989 Jul
	NTR-OR	1995 Oct
	NTR-OR	1997 Apr
2. Wasting diseases of teeth	NTR-NR	1997 Oct
3. Physiologic tooth mobility	NTR-NR	1990 Jul
4. Tooth mobility tests?	NTR-OR	1989 Jul

Brief notes

1. Tension test?	NTR-NR	2005 Apr
2. Tooth mobility?	NTR-NR	2006 Oct
3. Transgingival probing?	NTR-NR	2005 Oct
4. Causes and measurements of tooth mobility?	NTR-NR	2006 Oct

37. Radiographic Aids in the Diagnosis of the Periodontal Disease

Long essays

1. Define diagnosis. Describe the various microbiological investigations used in periodontal diagnosis. Add a note on the limitations of the radiographs in periodontal diagnosis?	NTR-NR	2003 Apr

Shanti

Short notes

1. Roentgenograms in periodontal diagnosis? NTR-OR 1992 Nov
2. Importance of radiographs in periodontics? NTR-OR 1998 Apr

Brief notes

38. Advanced Diagnostic Techniques

Long essays

Short notes

Brief notes

1. Periotemp NTR-NR 2005 Mar
2. DNA Probe NTR-NR 2002 Oct 252
   NTR-NR 2005 Mar

39. Risk Assessment

Long essays

Short notes

Brief notes

40. Levels of Clinical Significance

Long essays

Short notes

Brief notes

41. Determination of Prognosis

Long essays

1. Define prognosis. Describe in detail the various factors you consider to assess the prognosis NTR-NR 1997 Apr 237
2. Define prognosis. Write in detail the procedures adopted to assess the prognosis for periodontal treatment NTR-NR 1992 Oct 237
3. Define prognosis and discuss the various aspects which influences the prognosis of periodontal therapy NTR-NR 1989 Jul 237
4. Define prognosis what factors would you consider for determining the prognosis of a tooth with periodontal disease NTR-NR 1992 Nov 237

			Shanti
5. Define prognosis. Write in detail the procedure adopted to assess the prognosis for periodontal treatment?	NTR-OR	1999 Oct	237
6. What do you understand by the term prognosis? Enumerate the various factors which determine the prognosis of various factors which determine the prognosis of periodontal involved teeth	NTR-NR	1988 Jan	237

Short notes

1. Overall prognosis	NTR-NR	1998 Apr	238

Brief notes

42. The Treatment Plan

Long essays

Short notes

1. Phase 1 therapy?	NTR-NR	2005 Apr	256
2. Maintenance phase?	NTR-NR	2002 Oct	
	NTR-NR	2004 Apr	
3. Importance of maintenance phase?	NTR-OR	1996 Apr	

Brief notes

43. Rationale of Periodontal Treatment

Long essays

Short notes

Brief notes

44. Periodontal Therapy in the Female Patient

Long essays

Short notes

1. Periodontal therapy for pregnant patients?	NTR-NR	2005 Oct	119

Brief notes

45. Periodontal Treatment of Medically Compromised Patients

Long essays

1. Antibiotic prophylaxis for the medically compromised patients	NTR-NR	2005 Apr	

Short notes

Brief notes

46. Periodontal Treatment for Older Adults

Long essays

Short notes

Brief notes

47. Treatment for Aggressive and Atypical Forms of Periodontitis

Long essays

Short notes

Brief notes

48. Treatment of Acute Gingival Disease

Long essays

Short notes

1. Treatment of ANUG	NTR-OR	1996 Apr	170
	NTR-OR	1997 Oct	

Brief notes

49. Treatment of the Periodontal Abscess

Long essays

Short notes

1. Periodontal abscess	NTR-NR	1992 Nov	153
	NTR-OR	1998 Apr	
	NTR-OR	1999 Apr	
	NTR-NR	2004 Apr	

Brief notes

1. Periodontal abscess?	NTR-NR	2002 Oct	153
2. Difference between periodontal and periapical abscess?	NTR-NR	2000 Apr	

50. Phase I Periodontal Therapy

Long essays

1. What is Phase I therapy? Discuss the Importance	NTR-NR	1994 Nov	256

Shanti

Short notes

1. Phase I therapy	NTR-NR	2005 Apr	256

Brief notes

51. Plaque Control for the Periodontal Patient

Long essays

1. Describe the various methods of plaque control	NTR-NR	1995 Apr	280
2. What is plaque control? Describe the various aids used for interdental cleaning	NTR-NR	1993 May	280
3. What do you understand by plaque control and discuss the various interdental clearing aids?	NTR-OR	1995 Oct	280

Short notes

1. Dentifrice	NTR-NR	1998 Oct	284
	NTR-OR	2000 Apr	
2. Tooth brush	NTR-NR	2004 Oct	280
3. Dental floss	NTR-NR	1994 Nov	285
	NTR-OR	1996 Apr	
	NTR-OR	1999 Oct	
	NTR-OR	2001 Apr	
	NTR-NR	2006 Apr	
4. Ideal tooth brush	NTR-NR	1998 Oct	280
5. Interdental cleaners	NTR-NR	2004 Apr	285
6. Interdental devices?	NTR-OR	1989 Jan	285
7. Interdental cleaning aids	NTR-NR	1988 Jan	285
	NTR-OR	1990 Jul	
	NTR-NR	2002 Apr	
8. Interdental hygiene aids?	NTR-OR	1990 Jul	285
9. Disclosing solution	NTR-NR	2000 Apr	289
	NTR-NR	2001 Apr	
	NTR-NR	2006 Oct	
10. Desensitizing agents	NTR-NR	1994 May	
	NTR-OR	1995 Oct	
11. Chemical plaque control	NTR-NR	1994 May	286
12. Chlorhexidine?	NTR-OR	1988 Jan	340
	NTR-OR	2001 Oct	
13. Chlorhexidine-di-gluconate	NTR-NR	2002 Apr	340
14. Bass technique of tooth brushing	NTR-NR	2001 Oct	332
15. Uses and abuses of tooth brush	NTR-NR	1992 Nov	332
16. Chemical anti-plaque agents	NTR-OR	1996 Apr	338
17. Dental floss and technique of flossing	NTR-NR	2005 Oct	285

18. ADA specifications of a tooth brush	NTR-NR	2002 Oct	331
	NTR-NR	2004 Apr	
19. Oral prophylaxis and physiotherapy	NTR-OR	1983 Jul	

Brief notes

52. Scaling and Root Planning and Instrumentation

Long essays

1. Classify periodontal instruments and describe any one of them in detail	NTR-NR	1999 Apr	262
2. Describe the general principles you follow during oral prophylaxis?	NTR-OR	1998 Apr	269

Short notes

1. Finger rest	NTR-NR	2005 Apr	272
2. Naber's probe	NTR-NR	1998 Oct	
3. Kirkland knife	NTR-NR	1999 Oct	268
	NTR-NR	2001 Oct	
4. Periodontal probes	NTR-OR	1994 Nov	263
	NTR-OR	1997 Apr	
	NTR-OR	2000 Apr	
	NTR-NR	2001 Oct	
	NTR-NR	2006 Apr	
5. Polishing instruments	NTR-NR	1999 Apr	267
6. Area specific curettes?	NTR-NR	2005 Oct	265
7. Sharpening of periodontal instruments	NTR-OR	1996 Apr	269
	NTR-OR	1998 Apr	
8. Differences between scalers and curette?	NTR-OR	2000 Apr	

Brief notes

1. Gracey currets?	NTR-NR	2006 Apr	265

53. Chemotherapeutic Agents

Long essays

Short notes

1. Antibiotics	NTR-NR	1992 Nov	404
2. Periodontal pack?	NTR-OR	1989 Jan	125
	NTR-OR	1992 Nov	
	NTR-OR	1998 Apr	
3. Periodontal dressing?	NTR-OR	1993 May	125
	NTR-OR	1995 Apr	
	NTR-OR	1996 Apr	
	NTR-NR	2005 Apr	

4. Desensitizing agents?	NTR-OR	1994 May	
	NTR-OR	1995 Oct	
	NTR-NR	2006 Apr	405
5. Tetracyclines in periodontics?	NTR-NR	2004 Oct	408
6. Local drug delivery system?	NTR-NR	2005 Oct	
	NTR-NR	2006 Apr	
7. Antibiotic prophylaxis for the medically compromised patients?	NTR-NR	2005 Apr	

Brief notes

1. Periodontal dressing?	NTR-NR	2004 May	125
2. Desensitizing agents?	NTR-NR	2006 Apr	

54. Host Modulating Agents

Long essays

Short notes

Brief notes

55. Sonic and Ultrasonic Instrumentation

Long essays

Short notes

1. Ultrasonics	NTR-NR	1998 Apr	277
2. Ultrasonic scaling?	NTR-OR	1988 Jan	277
3. Ultrasonic scaler?	NTR-NR	2001 Oct	277
4. Ultrasonics in periodontics?	NTR-NR	2005 Oct	277

Brief notes

56. Supragingival and Subgingival Irrigation

Long essays

Short notes

Brief notes

57. Occlusal Evaluation and Therapy

Long essays

Short notes

1. Coronoplasty	NTR-NR	1994 Nov	379
	NTR-OR	1998 Oct	
	NTR-NR	2005 Oct	

2. Occlusal interferences?	NTR-OR	1995 Apr	394
3. Indications for occlusal adjustments?	NTR-OR	1992 Nov	395

Brief notes

1. Facets?	NTR-NR	2000 Apr	
	NTR-NR	2004 May	
2. Supracontacts?	NTR-NR	2006 Apr	
3. Occlusal adjustments?	NTR-NR	2000 Apr	395
4. Indications for coronoplasty?	NTR-NR	2002 Oct	395

58. Adjunctive Role of Orthodontic Therapy

Long essays

Short notes

Brief notes

59. The Periodontic–Endodontic Continuum

Long essays

Short notes

1. Retrograde periodontitis	NTR-NR	1997 Apr	373

Brief notes

60. Phase II Periodontal Therapy

Long essays

Short notes

Brief notes

61. General Principles of Periodontal Surgery

Long essays

1. Describe the concept of physiological tissue formation as an essential aspect of periodontal surgery?	NTR-OR	1997 Apr	

Short notes

1. Periodontal pack	NTR-NR	1989 Jan	294
	NTR-OR	1992 Nov	
	NTR-OR	1998 Apr	

Shanti

2. Periodontal dressing	NTR-OR	1993 May	294
	NTR-OR	1996 Apr	
	NTR-NR	2005 Apr	
3. Suture material used in periodontal surgery?	NTR-OR	1999 Apr	292

Brief notes

62. Surgical Anatomy of the Periodontium and Related Structures

Long essays

Short notes

1. Inverse Bevel incision	NTR-NR	1994 May	317
2. Reverse Bevel Incision	NTR-NR	1993 Oct	317
	NTR-OR	1995 Oct	
3. Papilla preservation flap	NTR-NR	2005 Apr	318

Brief notes

63. Gingival Curettage

Long essays

1. Define curettage and describe the indications and technique of subgingival curettage	NTR-NR	2000 Apr	303
2. Enumerate various gingival surgeries. Describe about any one of them?	NTR-OR	1983 Jul	

Short notes

1. ENAP	NTR-NR	1994 Nov	304
	NTR-OR	1997 Apr	
2. Gingival Curettage	NTR-NR	1992 Nov	
	NTR-OR	1993 Oct	303
	NTR-OR	2000 Apr	
3. Excisional new attachment procedure (ENAP)	NTR-NR	2005 Apr	304

Brief notes

1. Curettage?	NTR-NR	2004 May	303

64. Gingival Surgical Techniques

Long essays

1. Describe the surgical technique of gingivectomy	NTR-NR	1996 Apr	308
2. Write indications, disadvantages and step-by-step procedure of gingivectomy?	NTR-NR	2006 Oct	307
3. Discuss the step by step procedure of gingivectomy and mention on its indications and contraindications	NTR-NR	1989 Jan	308

Short notes

1. Gingivoplasty	NTR-OR	1988 Jan	307
	NTR-OR	1993 Aug	
	NTR-OR	1993 Oct	
	NTR-NR	2001 Apr	
2. Healing following gingivectomy	NTR-NR	1992 Nov	310
3. Indications of gingivectomy?	NTR-NR	2003 Apr	307
4. Healing of wound following Gingivectomy	NTR-NR	1995 Oct	310

Brief notes

65. Treatment of Gingival Enlargements

Long essays

Short notes

Brief notes

66. The Periodontal Flap

Long essays

1. Define and classify periodontal flap. Discuss the modified Widman's flap in detail	NTR-NR	2004 Oct	314
2. Classify periodontal pocket? Describe the nonsurgical treatment regimen which will help in pocket eliminating	NTR-NR	1988 Jan	
3. Define and classify flaps. Describe in detail the modifies Widman's flap technique	NTR-NR	2002 Oct	315

Short notes

1. Laterally repositioned flap?	NTR-OR	1988 Jan	352

Brief notes

67. The Flap Technique for the Pocket Therapy

Long essays

Short notes

1. Papilla preservation flap?	NTR-NR	2005 Apr	316

Brief notes

68. Resective Osseous Surgery

Long essays

Shanti

Short notes

1. Resective osseous surgery	NTR-OR	1998 Oct	330
2. Accordion technique?	NTR-OR	1994 Nov	346
3. Root surface bio-modification?	NTR-NR	2006 Apr	336
4. Difference between ostectomy and osteoplasty	NTR-NR	2002 Apr	330

Brief notes

1. Steps in resective osseous surgery	NTR-NR	2002 Apr	332

69. Reconstructive Periodontal Surgery

Long essays

1. Enumerate the various types of bone grafts and briefly on any one of them.	NTR-OR	1989 Jan	336
2. Define osseous surgery. Discuss various osseous grafting procedures?	NTR-NR	2005 Apr	336
3. Define repair and regeneration, enumerate the various regenerative treatment procedures Explain GTR procedure in detail	NTR-NR	2002 Apr	334

Short notes

1. Alloplast	NTR-NR	1994 Nov	338
	NTR-NR	2006 Oct	
2. Bone blend	NTR-NR	1995 Apr	338
3. Bone grafts?	NTR-NR	2004 May	337
4. New attachment?	NTR-OR	2000 Apr	259
5. Hydroxyapatite?	NTR-NR	2001 Apr	203
6. Osseous coagulum	NTR-NR	1994 May	337
	NTR-OR	1999 Oct	
7. Non-bone graft materials	NTR-NR	1998 Apr	338
8. Root treatment?	NTR-OR	2000 Apr	336
9. Reattachment?	NTR-OR	1983 Jul	259
10. Guided tissue regeneration	NTR-NR	1994 May	334
	NTR-NR	2003 Oct	
11. Guided tissue regeneration (GTR)	NTR-NR	2005 Oct	334

Brief notes

1. Root conditioning	NTR-NR	2004 Oct	336
2. Osseo integration?	NTR-NR	2005 Apr	381
	NTR-NR	2006 Oct	
3. Long Junctional epithelium?	NTR-NR	2005 Apr	260

70. Furcation Involvement and Treatment

Long essays

Question	University	Year	Page
1. What do you understand by furcation involvement? Give the etiology, classification and management of furcation involvement	NTR-NR	1992 Nov	365

Short notes

Question	University	Year	Page
1. Redirection	NTR-NR	1999 Apr	
2. Tunneling	NTR-NR	2001 Apr	369
3. Hemisection	NTR-OR	1989 Jan	370
	NTR-OR	1999 Oct	
	NTR-NR	2004 Oct	
	NTR-NR	2006 Oct	
4. Furcationplasty	NTR-NR	1990 Jul	
5. Tunneling procedure	NTR-NR	1995 Apr	369
6. Furcation involvement	NTR-NR	1998 Oct	365

Brief notes

Question	University	Year	Page
1. Classification of furcation involvement?	NTR-NR	2005 Apr	367

71. Periodontal Plastic and Esthetic Surgery

Long essays

Question	University	Year	Page
1. Enumerate the various gingival surgeries. Describe about any one of them.	NTR-OR	1988 Jul	
2. What is mucogingival surgery? Enumerate various mucogingival procedures. Add a note on Frenectomy?	NTR-OR	1994 May	341

Short notes

Question	University	Year	Page
1. Vestibuloplasty	NTR-NR	1993 May	348
	NTR-OR	1998 Apr	
	NTR-OR	2000 Apr	
2. Frenectomy	NTR-OR	1989 Jul	362
	NTR-OR	1995 Apr	
	NTR-OR	1997 Oct	
	NTR-NR	2004 Apr	
	NTR-NR	2005 Oct	
	NTR-NR	2006 Oct	
3. Frenectomy and Frenotomy?	NTR-NR	2003 Apr	362
4. High frenal attachment?	NTR-OR	1990 July	362
	NTR-OR	1999 Oct	

Brief notes

72. Recent Advances in Surgical Technology

Long essays

Short notes

Brief notes

73. Preparation of the Periodontium for the Restorative Dentistry

Long essays

Short notes

Brief notes

1. Biological width?	NTR-NR	2006 Apr	401

74. Periodontal Restorative Inter-relationships

Long essays

Short notes

1. Retrograde periodontitis?	NTR-OR	1997 Apr	373

Brief notes

75. Biologic Aspects of Dental Implants

Long essays

Short notes

Brief notes

76. Clinical Aspects and Evaluation of Implant Patient

Long essays

Short notes

Brief notes

77. Diagnostic Imaging for the Implant Patient

Long essays

Short notes

Brief notes

78. Standard Implant Surgical Procedures

Long essays

1. Define and classify implant material, add a note on the utility of implant material in periodontal therapy? NTR-OR 1990 Jul 381

Short notes

Brief notes

79. Localized Bone Augmentation and Implant Site Development

Long essays

Short notes

Brief notes

80. Advanced Implant Surgical Procedures

Long essays

Short notes

Brief notes

81. Recent Advances in Implant Surgical Technology

Long essays

Short notes

Brief notes

82. Biomechanics, Treatment Planning and Prosthetic Considerations

Long essays

Short notes

Brief notes

83. Implant-related Complications and Failures

Long essays

Short notes

Brief notes

84. Supportive Periodontal Treatment

Long essays

Short notes

1. Maintenance phase	NTR-NR	2004 Apr
2. Importance of maintenance phase	NTR-NR	1996 Apr
3. Supportive periodontal therapy?	NTR-NR	2006 Apr

Brief notes

85. Results of Periodontal Treatment

Long essays

Short notes

Brief notes

86. Dental Ethics

Long essays

Short notes

Brief notes

87. Legal Principles: Jurisprudence

Long essays

Short notes

Brief notes

88. Dental Insurance and Managed Care in Periodontal Practice

Long essays

Short notes

Brief notes

89. Principles of Research Methodology

Long essays

Short notes

Brief notes

Shanti

90. Research-related Periodontitis in Animals

Long essays

Short notes

Brief notes

91. Recent Concepts of Microbiology of Periodontitis in Man

Long essays

Short notes

Brief notes

92. Case History and Analysis Chart

Long essays

Short notes

Brief notes

93. Infection Control in Periodontics

Long essays

Short notes

Brief notes

94. Role of Computers in Periodontics

Long essays

Short notes

Brief notes

95. Splints in Periodontal Therapy

Long essays

1. Define and describe various splints	NTR-NR	1983 Jul	378

Short notes

1. Splinting	NTR-NR	1999 Apr	378
2. Periodontal splints?	NTR-NR	2006 Oct	378

Brief notes

1. Define and classify splints	NTR-NR	2002 Oct	378
2. Classification of periodontal splints?	NTR-NR	2005 Oct	378

96. Miscellaneous Topics

Long essays

1. "Periodontal health for all by 2000 AP" What do you understand by this statement. How are you going to implement it by systemic manner	NTR-NR	1997 Oct
2. Describe the concept of physiological tissue formation as an essential aspect of periodontal surgery?	NTR-OR	1997 Apr

Short notes

1. Biopsy?	NTR-OR	1997 Oct
2. Arthus reaction?	NTR-OR	1997 Oct
3. Incubation zone?	NTR-OR	1989 Jul
4. Embrassure forms	NTR-NR	2002 Apr
5. Desensitizing agents?	NTR-OR	1994 May
6. Inverse bevel incision?	NTR-OR	1994 May
7. Dentine hypersensitivity?	NTR-NR	2004 Apr
8. Benign tumors of gingiva?	NTR-OR	1995 Oct
9. Wasting diseases of teeth?	NTR-NR	2006 Apr
10. Feulgen positive particles?	NTR-OR	1989 Jul
11. Management of operative bleeding?	NTR-OR	2000 Apr
12. Inter-dental denudation procedure?	NTR-OR	1995 Apr

Brief notes

1. Periotemp?	NTR-NR	2005 Apr
	NTR-NR	2006 Oct
2. Periodontal disease activity?	NTR-NR	2005 Oct

OPERATIVE DENTISTRY

SYLLABUS

Examination

- Diagnosis and treatment planning.

Infection Control

- As related to conservative dentistry and endodontics
- Methods of sterilization of instruments, equipment's and materials
- Isolation of operating field
- Control of pain during operative procedures.

Instruments used in Conservative Dentistry

- Hand cutting instruments: Classification, instrument formula, Description of hand cutting instruments
- Rotary cutting instruments: Dental burs, classification of speeds
- Advantages and disadvantages of low and high speed
- Matrices and retainers used in restorative dentistry
- Separation of teeth
- Management of gingival tissue during operative procedures
- Contacts and contours.

Various Cavity Designs for Amalgam Restorations

- Restoration, finishing and polishing
- Pin retained amalgam restorations
- Bonded amalgam restorations
- Mercury hygiene.

Cast Gold Restoration

- Definitions of inlay and onlay
- Indications and contraindications
- Cavity designs for class II category gold inlay restorations wax patterns
- Spruing, investing and casting
- Seating, adjusting and polishing of the casting
- Cementation, Burnishing
- Casting defects, causes and prevention.

Direct Filling Gold Indication, Contraindication

- Various cavity designs and preparation of cavities
- Cohesive gold
- Principles of manipulation
- Compaction techniques, finishing and polishing.

Introduction Properties

- Indication of esthetic materials
- Acid etching technique–Enamel/Dentin in bonding system
- Tooth preparation, Restorative techniques

- Finishing and polishing procedures
- Glass ionomer restorations
- Clinical indications and contraindications
- Tooth preparation and manipulation
- Matrices, finishing and polishing procedures
- Recent advances in Glass ionomer cements
- Light cured composite inlay
- Veneers
- Hypersensitivity of teeth and management
- Pulpal reaction/response to various materials and procedures
- Diagnosis of dental caries and preventive restorative treatment.

Non-carious Lesions

- Attrition, Abrasion, Erosion
- Management.

Ceramic Restorations

- Ceramic inlays and onlay
- Clinical procedures for cerac-CAD/CAM
- Inlay and onlay.

Miscellaneous

- Laser
- Air abrasion
- Caries detector.

SCHEME OF EXAMINATION

Theory

Theory	–	70 Marks
Viva Voce	–	10 Marks
Internal Assessment (Theory)	–	20 Marks

Operative Dentistry (Part-A + Part-B / 35 + 35 = 70)

Subject	*Type of question*	*Marks offered*	*Total*
Part-A/Operative Dentistry	Long essays	9	1 x 9 = 09
	Short notes	4	4 x 4 = 16
	Brief notes	2	5 x 2 = 10
Part-B/Operative Dentistry	Long essays	9	1 x 9 = 09
	Short notes	4	4 x 4 = 16
	Brief notes	2	5 x 2 = 10

Clinicals

Clinicals	–	70 Marks
Viva Voce	–	10 Marks
Internal Assessment (Clinicals)	–	20 Marks

REFERENCE BOOK

Operative Dentistry: Textbook of Operative Dentistry – By Narendranath Reddy

AUTHOR ABBREVIATION

Narendra: Narendranath Reddy

Edition: 2nd

QUESTION BANK ABBREVIATION

Question Bank

LE — Long essays
SN — Short notes
BN — Brief notes

University

NTRUHS — Nandamuri Taraka Rama Rao University of Health Sciences
NTRUHS-NR — NTRUHS–New Regulations
NTRUHS-OR — NTRUHS–Old Regulations

CONTENTS

OPERATIVE DENTISTRY

Narendra

1. History of Operative Dentistry

Long essays

Short notes

Brief notes

2. Fundamental Concepts of Operative Dentistry

Long essays

Short notes

Brief notes

3. Occlusion

Long essays

Short notes

Brief notes

4. Cariology: Dental Caries

Long essays

Short notes

1. Caries activity tests?	NTR-NR	2006 Apr	45
2. Classification of dental caries?	NTR-NR	2001 Apr	43

Brief notes

5. Non-carious Lesions

Long essays

1. Describe the technique of restoring an abrasive lesion in an upper first premolar?	NTR-OR	1997 Oct	138

Narendra

Short notes

1. Microabrasion?	NTR-NR	2005 Apr	144
2. Causes of wasting diseases of teeth?	NTR-NR	2005 Oct	137

Brief notes

1. Abfraction?	NTR-NR	2004 Oct	113
2. Abrasion?	NTR-NR	2006 Oct	138
3. Macroabrasion?	NTR-NR	2005 Oct	144

6. Dentin Hypersensitivity

Long essays

1. Discuss etiology and management of hypersensitive dentine?	NTR-OR	1999 Oct	140

Short notes

1. Management of hypersensitive dentine?	NTR-NR	2002 Apr	141
	NTR-NR	2004 Apr	
	NTR-NR	2004 Oct	
	NTR-NR	2005 Mar	

Brief notes

1. Causes of dentine hypersensitivity?	NTR-NR	2006 Apr	140

7. Biological Considerations in Restorative Dentistry

Long essays

Short notes

1. Secondary dentin	NTR-NR	2002 Apr	152

Brief notes

1. Secondary dentin?	NTR-NR	2004 Apr	152

8. Periodontal Aspects of Restorative Dentistry

Long essays

Short notes

Brief notes

9. Diagnosis and Treatment Planning

Long essays

Short notes

Brief notes

10. Operative Dentistry Armamentarium

Long essays

1. Classify speeds in dentistry. Write in detail the advantages of High-speed diagnosis ultra high speed in dental practice?	NTR-OR	1991 Mar	57

Short notes

1. Instrument formula?	NTR-NR	2002 Oct	52
	NTR-OR	1992 Nov	
2. Instrument formula for hand cutting instruments?	NTR-OR	1999 Oct	52
3. Finger rests and guards?	NTR-OR	1992 Nov	56
4. Angle former?	NTR-NR	2002 Apr	55
5. Enamel Hatchet?	NTR-OR	1995 Oct	55
	NTR-OR	1997 Oct	
6. Hatchet and Hoe?	NTR-NR	2000 Apr	55
7. Amalgam Carver?	NTR-NR	2002 Apr	63
8. Marginal trimmers?	NTR-OR	1993 May	55
9. Gingival Marginal trimmer?	NTR-OR	1994 Nov	55
	NTR-NR	2001 Oct	
10. High speed?	NTR-OR	1998 Oct	62
11. Ultra speed?	NTR-NR	2004 Oct	62
12. Advantages and disadvantages of high speed?	NTR-OR	1997 Apr	62
	NTR-NR	2002 Apr	
13. Rotatory cutting instrument?	NTR-NR	2006 Oct	57
14. Dental burs?	NTR-OR	1998 Apr	58
	NTR-NR	2004 May	
15. Bur design?	NTR-NR	2005 Apr	59

Brief notes

1. Slow speed?	NTR-NR	2006 Oct	62
2. Gingival marginal trimmers?	NTR-NR	2006 Apr	55

11. Matrices, Wedges and Retainers

Long essays

Short notes

1. Matrices?	NTR-OR	1999 Apr	82
	NTR-NR	2005 Oct	

			Narendra
2. Tofflemier matrix retainers?	NTR-NR	2002 Apr	83
3. Matrices and retainers used in restorative dentistry?	NTR-NR	2000 Apr	82

Brief notes

1. Wedge?	NTR-NR	2006 Apr	84
2. Tofflemier retainers?	NTR-NR	2006 Oct	83

12. Contacts and Contours

Long essays

1. How will you gain the active separation of teeth in operative dentistry?	NTR-OR	1992 Apr	81

Short notes

1. Separators?	NTR-OR	1991 Mar	81
	NTR-NR	2005 Apr	
2. Mechanical separators?	NTR-OR	1993 May	81
3. Contacts and contours?	NTR-NR	2001 Oct	81
4. Separation of teeth?	NTR-OR	1997 Oct	80
	NTR-OR	1999 Oct	

Brief notes

1. Separators?	NTR-NR	2005 Apr	81
2. Embrasures?	NTR-NR	2002 Oct	79
	NTR-NR	2004 Apr	
3. Elliot separator?	NTR-NR	2004 Apr	81
4. Significance of contacts and contours?	NTR-NR	2006 Apr	80

13. Isolation of the Operating Field

Long essays

1. Discuss the importance of isolation of the operating field and various methods to achieve it in conservative dentistry?	NTR-NR	2005 Oct	69

Short notes

1. Rubber dam?	NTR-OR	1992 Nov	71
2. Retraction Chord?	NTR-NR	2001 Apr	70
3. Management of Rubber dam	NTR-NR	1992 Nov	71
4. Describe components of Rubber dam kit?	NTR-NR	2001 Apr	71
5. Gingival retraction?	NTR-OR	1993 May	70
	NTR-OR	1997 Apr	
	NTR-OR	1998 Oct	
6. Gingival tissue management?	NTR-OR	1991 Mar	70

7. Management of gingival tissues during operative procedures?	NTR-NR	2004 Oct	70

Brief notes

1. Gingival retraction?	NTR-NR	2005 Oct	70
2. Advantages off rubber dam?	NTR-NR	2005 Oct	71

14. Principles of Cavity Preparation

Long essays

1. Give GV Black's classification of cavities?	NTR-OR	1995 Oct	45
2. Describe briefly modern method of class II cavity preparation. Please also mention modification in this from GV Black principles?	NTR-OR	1991 Mar	10, 45

Short notes

1. Outline form?	NTR-NR	2006 Apr	10
2. Retention form?	NTR-OR	1995 Oct	11

Brief notes

1. Reverse curve?	NTR-NR	2005 Oct	92
	NTR-NR	2006 Oct	
2. Convience form?	NTR-NR	2004 Oct	11
	NTR-NR	2005 Oct	
3. External outline form?	NTR-NR	2006 Oct	10

15. Interim Restorative Materials

Long essays

Short notes

1. Silicate cement?	NTR-OR	1995 Oct	99
2. Zinc phosphate cement?	NTR-OR	1992 Apr	26
3. Zinc poly carboxylate cement?	NTR-OR	1998 Oct	25
4. Modified zinc oxide eugenol cement?	NTR-OR	1994 Nov	26
5. Uses of zinc oxide eugenol cement?	NTR-NR	2006 Apr	26
6. Intermediate restorative materials?	NTR-OR	1995 Apr	32

Brief notes

16. Silver Amalgam Restorations

Long essays

1. Define cavity preparation. Describe the outline form for silver amalgam restoration?	NTR-OR	1995 Oct	86

Narendra

2. Describe class II cavity preparation for silver amalgam with emphasis on modern concepts?	NTR-OR	1998 Apr	89
3. Define retention and resistance form. Describe the technique of obtaining the same for the class II cavity for silver amalgam?	NTR-NR	2001 Oct	88
4. Write in detail the class II cavity preparation for silver amalgam restoration and a not an usage of Hand cutting instruments?	NTR-OR	1998 Oct	88
5. Describe the technique of class II cavity preparation for silver amalgam in an upper first molar. Mention the advantages of High copper amalgam?	NTR-NR	2004 Oct	88
6. Describe the technique of class II cavity preparations for silver amalgam in mandibular 1st molar?	NTR-OR	1992 Nov	88
7. Write differences in Class II cavity for silver amalgam and gold inlay?	NTR-NR	2002 Apr	88

Short notes

1. Retention for silver amalgam?	NTR-OR	1992 Nov	89
2. High copper amalgam?	NTR-OR	1990 Feb	17
	NTR-OR	1990 Oct	
	NTR-OR	1997 Oct	
	NTR-OR	1999 Apr	
	NTR-NR	2000 Apr	
	NTR-NR	2006 Oct	
3. Advantages of High copper amalgam?	NTR-NR	2002 Oct	17
4. Metallurgy of silver amalgam?	NTR-NR	2005 Oct	17
5. Mercuroscopic expansion?	NTR-OR	1995 Oct	
6. Delayed expansion of amalgam?	NTR-OR	1998 Oct	23
7. Mercury hygiene?	NTR-OR	1997 Apr	23
	NTR-NR	2004 Apr	
8. Mercury toxicity?	NTR-NR	2006 Apr	23

Brief notes

1. Eame's technique?	NTR-NR	2005 Apr	19

17. Pins in Restorative dentistry

Long essays

Short notes

1. TMS pins?	NTR-OR	1992 Nov	95
2. Self shearing pins?	NTR-OR	1998 Apr	95
	NTR-OR	2000 Apr	

			Narendra

Brief notes

1. Self shearing pins?	NTR-NR	2002 Oct	95

18. Direct Filling Gold Restoration

Long essays

Short notes

1. Indications for direct filling gold?	NTR-NR	2002 Apr	116
2. Compaction of direct filling gold?	NTR-NR	2001 Oct	118

Brief notes

19. Cast Metal Restorations

Long essays

1. What are the indications for gold inlay? Describe the cavity preparation for class II gold inlay in upper first molar?	NTR-NR	2004 Apr	129
2. Define Inlay. Describe the indications, contraindications, advantages and disadvantages of cast gold restorations?	NTR-OR	1995 Apr	133
3. Describe the class II cavity preparation for gold inlay and preparation of direct wax pattern?	NTR-OR	2000 Apr	133
4. Write in detail the class II cavity preparation for gold inlay and how do you proceed to take direct wax pattern?	NTR-OR	1999 Apr	129
5. Give indications for gold inlay. Describe the differences in cavity preparations between silver amalgam and gold inlay?	NTR-OR	1997 Apr	129
6. Write differences in class II cavity for silver amalgam and gold inlay?	NTR-NR	2002 Apr	129, 132

Short notes

1. Bevels?	NTR-OR	1991 Mar	131
	NTR-NR	2002 Oct	
2. Beveling?	NTR-OR	1997 Apr	131
	NTR-OR	1998 Apr	
3. Cavity bevels?	NTR-OR	1994 Nov	131
4. Types of bevels?	NTR-NR	2005 Apr	131
5. Bevels in cavity preparation?	NTR-OR	1999 Oct	131
6. Indications for the gold inlay?	NTR-OR	1992 Apr	129

Brief notes

Narendra

20. Dental Casting Procedures

Long essays

No.	Question	University	Year	Page
1.	Enumerate the casting defects and discuss in detail?	NTR-OR	1994 Nov	39
2.	Describe briefly the methods used in compensating casting shrinkage of gold in casting procedures?	NTR-OR	1990 Feb	39

Short notes

No.	Question	University	Year	Page
1.	Sprue?	NTR-OR	1995 Oct	36
2.	Sprue former?	NTR-NR	2004 Oct	36
3.	Sprue & Sprue former?	NTR-NR	2005 Oct	36
4.	Casting Machines?	NTR-OR	1997 Oct	38
		NTR-NR	2001 Oct	
5.	Casting techniques?	NTR-OR	1991 Mar	39
6.	Porosities in castings?	NTR-OR	1998 Apr	39
7.	Porosities in dental castings?	NTR-OR	1999 Oct	39
8.	Subsurface porosity in gold alloy castings?	NTR-OR	1993 May	39
9.	Investment material?	NTR-OR	1995 Apr	38
10.	Gypsum bonded investment material?	NTR-OR	1992 Nov	38
11.	Inlay wax?	NTR-OR	1992 Apr	
		NTR-OR	1994 May	
		NTR-OR	1995 Apr	
12.	Advantages and disadvantages indirect wax pattern?	NTR-OR	1994 Nov	36
13.	Advantages and disadvantages of direct wax pattern?	NTR-OR	1992 Apr	36

Brief notes

21. Composite Resin Restorations

Long essays

No.	Question	University	Year	Page
1.	Discuss status of composite resins as a posterior restorative material?	NTR-NR	2005 Apr	102
2.	Give indications for composite resins. Describe the procedure of restoring fractured incisal angle?	NTR-NR	2002 Oct	100

Short notes

No.	Question	University	Year	Page
1.	Percolation?	NTR-OR	1998 Oct	
2.	Inactivators?	NTR-OR	1995 Oct	
3.	Acid etching?	NTR-OR	1998 Apr	103
		NTR-NR	2000 Apr	
4.	Direct composite veneers?	NTR-NR	2006 Apr	102
5.	Bilayered technique?	NTR-NR	2004 Apr	114
6.	Acid etching on enamel?	NTR-OR	1999 Apr	103
7.	Visible light cured composites?	NTR-NR	2004 Oct	102
8.	Types of fillers used in composite resins?	NTR-OR	Oct 1999	

Brief notes

Narendra

22. Bonding and Bonding Agents

Long essays

Short notes

1. Bonding agents?	NTR-OR	1997 Apr	104
2. Dentine bonding?	NTR-NR	2002 Apr	104
3. Dentine bonding agents?	NTR-OR	1999 Oct	104
	NTR-NR	2001 Oct	
	NTR-NR	2004 May	
4. Lasers in dentistry?	NTR-NR	2006 Oct	144

Brief notes

1. Lasers?	NTR-NR	2004 May	144
2. Smear layer?	NTR-NR	2002 Oct	104
	NTR-NR	2004 Oct	

23. Glass Ionomer Cement

Long essays

1. Describe merits and demerits of glass ionomer cement diagnosis applications in restorative dentistry?	NTR-NR	2001 Apr	110

Short notes

1. Hybrid Ionomer?	NTR-OR	1998 Apr	30
	NTR-OR	2000 Apr	
2. Glass cerment cements?	NTR-OR	1993 May	29
3. Glass Ionomer cement?	NTR-OR	1990 Feb	29
	NTR-OR	1992 Nov	
4. Type II Glass Ionomer cement?	NTR-OR	1999 Apr	29

Brief notes

24. Dental Ceramics

Long essays

Short notes

1. Veneers?	NTR-NR	2001 Apr	111

Brief notes

25. Color and Its Applications

Long essays

Short notes

Brief notes

26. Cervical Lesions

Long essays

Short notes

Brief notes

1.	Abfraction?	NTR-NR	2004 Oct	113

27. Finishing and Polishing

Long essays

Short notes

1.	Finishing of gold Inlay?	NTR-OR	1992 Nov	135
2.	Finishing and polishing of silver amalgam?	NTR-OR	1992 Apr	93
3.	Finishing and polishing of amalgam restoration?	NTR-NR	2001 Apr	93

Brief notes

28. Micro Leakage

Long essays

Short notes

Brief notes

29. Biocompatible Aspects of Restorative Materials

Long essays

Short notes

Brief notes

30. Preventive Measures in Restorative Dentistry

Long essays

Short notes

1.	Prophylactic ododntotomy?	NTR-NR	2001 Apr

Brief notes

1.	Pit and fissure sealants?	NTR-NR	2005 Apr

31. Miscellaneous

Long essays

1.	Discuss control of pain during operative procedures?	NTR-NR	2006 Apr
2.	State various morphological defects of tooth structure. How will you treat them?	NTR-NR	2006 Oct

Narendra

3. Describe a method conservative restoration of fractured maxillary vital incisor teeth?	NTR-OR	1993 May	
4. Enumerate the various teeth colored restorative material. Give composition, manipulation, indications and advantages of silicate cement?	NTR-OR	1992 Apr	

Short notes

1. Plunger cusp?	NTR-NR	2002 Apr	32
2. Luting cements?	NTR-NR	2004 Oct	32
	NTR-NR	2006 Oct	
3. Cavity liners?	NTR-OR	1997 Oct	31
4. Cavity varnish?	NTR-OR	1999 Apr	31
	NTR-NR	2002 Oct	
	NTR-NR	2005 Apr	
5. Cavity varnish and liners?	NTR-OR	1992 Apr	31
6. Slice preparation?	NTR-OR	1992 Apr	134
7. Tunnel preparation?	NTR-NR	2001 Oct	92
	NTR-NR	2002 Oct	
8. Circumferential tie?	NTR-NR	2005 Oct	205
9. Bilayered technique?	NTR-NR	2004 Apr	114
10. CAD-CAM?	NTR-NR	2004 Apr	143
11. Soldering?	NTR-OR	1992 Apr	
	NTR-OR	1999 Apr	
12. Tarnish and corrosion?	NTR-OR	1998 Oct	
13. Surface hardness?	NTR-OR	1995 Apr	
14. Dispersion alloy?	NTR-OR	1995 Apr	
15. Inactivators?	NTR-OR	1995 Oct	142
16. Lasers in dentistry?	NTR-NR	2006 Oct	

Brief notes

1. Post and core?	NTR-NR	2002 Oct
2. Phosphoric acid?	NTR-NR	2004 Oct

ENDODONTICS

SYLLABUS

1. Rationale of endodontic therapy.
2. Diagnostic aids in endodontics.
3. Care and sterilization of instruments for endodontics.
4. Treatment of vital and non-vital pulp.
5. Tests for sterility of the root canal.
6. Drugs used in the root canal therapy.
7. Bleaching of the teeth.
8. Restoration of the endodontically treated teeth.
9. Surgical treatment of endodontics.

SCHEME OF EXAMINATION

Theory

Theory – 70 Marks

Viva Voce – 10 Marks

Internal Assessment (Theory) – 20 Marks

Operative Dentistry (Part-A + Part-B / 35 + 35 = 70)

Subject	*Type of question*	*Marks offered*	*Total*
Part-A/Conservative Dentistry	Long essays	9	1 x 9 = 09
	Short notes	4	4 x 4 = 16
	Brief notes	2	5 x 2 = 10
Part-B/Endodontics	Long essays	9	1 x 9 = 09
	Short notes	4	4 x 4 = 16
	Brief notes	2	5 x 2 = 10

Clinicals

Clinicals – 70 Marks

Viva Voce – 10 Marks

Internal Assessment (Clinicals) – 20 Marks

REFERENCE BOOK

Endodontics: Textbook of Endodontics – By Narendranath Reddy

AUTHOR ABBREVIATION

Narendra: Narendranath Reddy

Edition: 2nd

QUESTION BANK ABBREVIATION

Question Bank

LE — Long essays
SN — Short notes
BN — Brief notes

University

NTRUHS — Nandamuri Taraka Rama Rao University of Health Sciences
NTRUHS-NR — NTRUHS–New Regulations
NTRUHS-OR — NTRUHS–Old Regulations

CONTENTS

ENDODONTICS

Narendra

1. Introduction to Endodontics

Long essays

Short notes

Brief notes

2. Endodontic Anatomy

Long essays

Short notes

1. Accessory canals?	NTR-NR	2001 Apr	154
2. Anatomy of root canal of maxillary permanent first molar?	NTR-NR	2005 Apr	156

Brief notes

1. C-shaped canal configuration?	NTR-NR	2006 Apr	

3. Diseases of the Dental Pulp and the Periapical Tissues

Long essays

Short notes

1. Pink tooth?	NTR-NR	2005 Apr	161
2. Anachoresis?	NTR-OR	1990 Feb	160
	NTR-OR	1992 Nov	
	NTR-OR	1994 Nov	
3. Reversible pulpitis?	NTR-OR	2000 Apr	160
4. Irreversible pulpitis?	NTR-OR	1998 Apr	160
5. Internal resorption?	NTR-NR	2004 Oct	161
	NTR-NR	2006 Oct	

Brief notes

1. Internal resorption?	NTR-NR	2006 Oct	161
2. Atrophy and fibrosis of pulp?	NTR-NR	2006 Apr	162
3. Calcific metamorphosis of pulp?	NTR-NR	2005 Oct	162

Narendra

4. Diseases of the Periradicular Tissues

Long essays

Short notes

1. Phoenix abscess?	NTR-OR	1997 Apr	165
	NTR-OR	1999 Oct	
	NTR-NR	2005 Oct	
2. Acute periapical abscess?	NTR-NR	2006 Apr	164

Brief notes

5. Endodontic Microbiology

Long essays

Short notes

1. Culture methods in endodontics?	NTR-NR	2006 Apr	168
2. Culture technique in endodontics?	NTR-OR	1991 Mar	168
	NTR-OR	1994 Nov	

Brief notes

1. Culture media used in endodontics?	NTR-NR	2004 Oct	168

6. Clinical Diagnostic Methods

Long essays

1. Describe the various diagnostic aids employed in endodontic practice?	NTR-OR	1992 Nov	170

Short notes

1. Pulp tests?	NTR-OR	1995 Apr	173
	NTR-OR	1998 Oct	
2. Test cavity?	NTR-OR	1995 Apr	175
	NTR-OR	1998 Apr	
3. Thermal test?	NTR-OR	1992 Apr	174
4. Vitality tests?	NTR-OR	1993 May	174
5. Electric pulp test?	NTR-OR	2000 Apr	172
6. Radiographic examination in endodontics?	NTR-OR	1994 Nov	172
7. Role of radiographs in endodontic practice?	NTR-OR	1995 Apr	172
	NTR-NR	2001 Apr	
8. False-positive and false-negative responses to electric pulp tester?	NTR-NR	2004 Oct	173

Brief notes

1. RVG?	NTR-NR	2004 Apr	202

			Narendra
2. Pulp vitality tests?	NTR-NR	2005 Oct	173
3. Importance of buccal-object rule in radiographs?	NTR-NR	2005 Oct	173

7. Sterilization in Endodontics

Long essays

1. Classify endodontic instruments and briefly describe the methods of sterilization of instrument?	NTR-OR	1998 Oct	176

Short notes

1. Hot salt sterilizer?	NTR-OR	1999 Oct	187
	NTR-NR	2001 Oct	
2. Glass bead sterilizer?	NTR-NR	2002 Oct	187
3. Asepsis in endodontics?	NTR-OR	1997 Oct	184
4. Sterilization of intra-canal instruments?	NTR-OR	1995 Apr	186

Brief notes

1. Disinfection?	NTR-NR	2005 Apr	208
2. Chemiclaving?	NTR-NR	2005 Apr	187

8. Endodontic Armamentarium

Long essays

1. Classify endodontic instruments and briefly describe the methods of sterilization of instrument?	NTR-OR	1998 Oct	176
2. Classification of endodontic instruments. Describe the hand instruments used for canal preparation?	NTR-NR	2002 Oct	176

Short notes

1. Endosonics?	NTR-OR	1993 May	183
	NTR-OR	1999 Oct	
2. Barbed broach?	NTR-OR	1994 Nov	178
	NTR-OR	1995 Oct	
3. Hedstrom files?	NTR-OR	1997 Oct	179
4. Endodontic files?	NTR-NR	2001 Apr	182
5. Gates-Glidden Drill?	NTR-OR	2000 Apr	182
	NTR-NR	2005 Oct	
6. Classification of endodontic instruments?	NTR-OR	1998 Apr	176
7. Standardization of root canal instruments?	NTR-OR	1997 Apr	177
8. Advantages and disadvantages of NITI rotatory endodontic instruments?	NTR-NR	2005 Oct	179

Brief notes

1. Endosonics?	NTR-NR	2004 Oct	183

				Narendra
2. Peeso reamers?	NTR-NR	2004 Apr	182	
3. Barbed broaches?	NTR-NR	2005 Apr	178	
4. Gates Glidden drills?	NTR-NR	2002 Oct	182	
	NTR-NR	2006 Apr		

9. Endodontic Materials

Long essays

1. Classify and describe the obturation materials and sealers used in root canal treatment?	NTR-NR	2001 Oct	212
2. Classify and describe the various intracanal medicaments in root canal treatment?	NTR-NR	2001 Apr	208
3. Mention the various irritants used in endodontics. Describe ideal properties and techniques of irrigation?	NTR-OR	1997 Apr	198

Short notes

1. MTA?	NTR-NR	2006 Oct	240
2. CMCP?	NTR-OR	1995 Oct	
3. EDTA?	NTR-OR	1997 Apr	199
	NTR-OR	1998 Apr	
	NTR-OR	1999 Oct	
4. Gutta-percha?	NTR-OR	1999 Apr	216
	NTR-NR	2001 Apr	
5. Thermoplasticized gutta-percha?	NTR-OR	1998 Apr	220
6. Root canal irrigants?	NTR-OR	1998 Oct	198
7. Bleaching agents?	NTR-OR	1994 Nov	
8. Sodium hypochlorite?	NTR-OR	1997 Oct	199
	NTR-NR	2001 Oct	
9. Intracanal medicaments?	NTR-OR	1999 Apr	208
10. Poly-antibiotic pastes?	NTR-OR	1992 Nov	209
11. Calcium hydroxide?	NTR-OR	2000 Apr	209
12. Uses of calcium hydroxide in endodontics?	NTR-OR	1997 Apr	209
13. Ideal requirements of root canal sealers?	NTR-NR	2004 Apr	212

Brief notes

1. Gutta-percha?	NTR-OR	1999 Apr	216
	NTR-NR	2001 Apr	
2. Glutaraldehyde?	NTR-NR	2004 Apr	209
3. Bleaching agents?	NTR-NR	2006 Oct	253
4. Sodium hypochlorite?	NTR-NR	2002 Oct	199
	NTR-NR	2004 Apr	
	NTR-NR	2006 Apr	
	NTR-NR	2006 Aug	
5. EDTA in endodontics?	NTR-NR	2005 Apr	199

			Narendra
6. Sodium hypochlorite solution?	NTR-OR	1995 Apr	199
7. Uses of $Ca(OH)_2$ in endodontics?	NTR-NR	2006 Oct	209
8. Role of $Ca(OH)_2$ in endodontics?	NTR-NR	2005 Oct	209
9. $Ca(OH)_2$ based root canal sealer?	NTR-NR	2001 Apr	209
10. Thermoplasticized gutta-percha?	NTR-OR	1998 Apr	211
	NTR-OR	1999 Oct	
11. Carbamide peroxide?	NTR-NR	2004 Oct	253
12. Gross man's sealers?	NTR-NR	2002 Oct	213
13. Uses of MTA in endodontics?	NTR-NR	2005 Oct	240

10. RCT: An Overview

Long essays

Short notes

Brief notes

11. Rationale of Endodontic Treatment

Long essays

1. Describe in detail rational of endodontic treatment?	NTR-OR	1990 Feb	189
2. Describe rationale and principles of endodontic treatment?	NTR-OR	1998 Apr	189
	NTR-OR	2000 Apr	

Short notes

1. Rational of endodontics?	NTR-NR	2004 Apr	189

Brief notes

12. Principle of Endodontic Treatment

Long essays

1. Describe the rationale and principles of endodontic treatment?	NTR-OR	1998 Apr	189
	NTR-OR	2000 Apr	

Short notes

Brief notes

13. Selection of Cases for Endodontic Treatment

Long essays

Short notes

Brief notes

14. Principles of Endodontic Cavity Preparation/Biomechanical Preparation

Long essays

1. Describe the biomechanical preparation in endodontics?	NTR-OR	1995 Apr	204

Short notes

1. Trephination?	NTR-OR	1993 May	185
	NTR-OR	1997 Apr	
	NTR-OR	1999 Apr	
	NTR-NR	2004 Apr	
2. Access cavity?	NTR-NR	2002 Oct	195
3. Access cavities in lower and upper molars?	NTR-OR	1990 Feb	196
4. Step back preparation?	NTR-OR	1993 May	205
	NTR-NR	2004 Apr	
5. Crown down pressure technique?	NTR-OR	2000 Apr	206

Brief notes

1. Access opening?	NTR-NR	2006 Oct	195
2. Recapitulation?	NTR-NR	2002 Oct	207
	NTR-NR	2004 Oct	
	NTR-NR	2005 Oct	

15. Working Length Determination

Long essays

1. What are the various methods of determining working length in endodontics?	NTR-OR	1990 Sep	200
2. What are the various methods of measuring the length of teeth in endodontics? Describe any one method?	NTR-OR	1991 Mar	200
	NTR-OR	1999 Oct	

Short notes

1. RVG in endodontics?	NTR-NR	2001 Oct	202
2. Ingle's method of determining working length?	NTR-NR	2002 Oct	201

Brief notes

1. RVG?	NTR-NR	2004 Apr	202
2. Apex locators?	NTR-NR	2005 Apr	

16. Disinfection of the Root Canal

Long essays

1. What do you understand by cleaning and shaping of root canal? Describe the instruments used for the same?	NTR-NR	2002 Oct	204

			Narendra

Short notes

1. Irrigation?	NTR-NR	2006 Apr	198
2. Irrigation in root canal therapy?	NTR-NR	2006 Oct	198

Brief notes

1. Disinfection?	NTR-NR	2005 Apr	208

17. Obturation of the Root Canal

Long essays

1. Classify and describe the obturation materials and sealers used in root canal treatment?	NTR-OR	2001 Oct	212
2. Classify obturating materials. Describe lateral condensation method of obturation of root canal?	NTR-NR	2002 Apr	215
3. Describe in detail lateral condensation – technique of root canal obturation?	NTR-OR	1993 May	218
4. How do you know that the root canal system is ready for obturation? Discuss lateral condensation technique?	NTR-NR	2005 Apr	215

Short notes

1. Crown down-pressure less technique?	NTR-OR	2000 Apr	206
2. Warm gutta-percha technique?	NTR-NR	2004 Oct	218
3. Thermoplastisized gutta-percha technique?	NTR-OR	1999 Oct	221

Brief notes

1. Schilder's technique?	NTR-NR	2006 Apr	218

18. Restoration of the Endodontically Treated Tooth

Long essays

1. Enumerate indications, contraindications and technique of post and core?	NTR-NR	2005 Oct	204

Short notes

Brief notes

19. Endodontic Procedural Mishaps

Long essays

1. Discuss in detail the sequale and treatment of incomplete root canal filling?	NTR-OR	1994 Nov	228

Short notes

Brief notes

Narendra

20. Failures of Endodontic Treatment

Long essays

1. Write various endodontic failures. How will you overcome them?	NTR-NR	2006 Oct	232

Short notes

Brief notes

21. Single-visit Endodontics

Long essays

Short notes

Brief notes

22. Bleaching of Discolored Teeth

Long essays

1. Mention the causes of discoloration of teeth	NTR-OR	1999 Apr	252
2. Mention the various cases for discoloration of teeth. Describe the techniques of bleaching vital discolored teeth?	NTR-NR	2004 Apr	252

Short notes

1. Walking bleach?	NTR-OR	1993 May	254
	NTR-OR	1998 Oct	
2. Night guard bleach?	NTR-OR	1997 Oct	255
	NTR-OR	1999 Oct	
3. Bleaching of discolored vital teeth?	NTR-OR	2001 Oct	254

Brief notes

1. Bleaching agents?	NTR-NR	2006 Oct	252
2. Causes of intrinsic discoloration of teeth?	NTR-NR	2006 Apr	252

23. Endodontic Emergencies

Long essays

Short notes

1. Phoenix abscess?	NTR-OR	1997 Apr	165
	NTR-OR	1999 Oct	

Brief notes

			Narendra

24. Pediatric Endodontics

Long essays

Short notes

1. Pulpotomy?	NTR-OR	1995 Oct	238
	NTR-OR	1999 Apr	
2. Pulp capping?	NTR-NR	2004 Apr	
3. Apexogensis?	NTR-OR	1995 Apr	242
4. Apexification?	NTR-OR	1990 Feb	241
	NTR-OR	1993 May	242
	NTR-OR	1995 Oct	
	NTR-OR	2001 Oct	
5. Apexification and Apexogensis?	NTR-NR	2005 Apr	241, 242
	NTR-NR	2006 Apr	

Brief notes

25. Treatment of Traumatized Teeth

Long essays

Short notes

Brief notes

26. Replantation, Transplantation and Endodontic Implants

Long essays

1. What is replantation? Write in detail intentional replantation?	NTR-OR	1991 Mar	248
2. Define intentional replantation. Write indications, contraindications and techniques of intentional replantation?	NTR-NR	2006 Apr	249

Short notes

1. Replantation?	NTR-OR	1998 Oct	249
2. Intentional replantation?	NTR-OR	1990 Feb	249
	NTR-OR	1998 Apr	
	NTR-NR	2006 Oct	
3. Replantation of avulsed tooth?	NTR-NR	2004 Oct	248
4. Endodontic implant?	NTR-OR	1992 Apr	250
5. Endodontic endosseous implants?	NTR-NR	2002 Oct	250

Brief notes

Narendra

27. Endodontic Surgeries

Long essays

Question	University	Year	Page
1. Give indications, for periapical surgery. Describe briefly the procedure of Apicoectomy in a maxillary central incisor?	NTR-OR	1997 Oct	259

Short notes

Question	University	Year	Page
1. Radisection?	NTR-OR	1999 Apr	262
2. Hemisection?	NTR-OR	1998 Oct	262
	NTR-NR	2001 Apr	
3. Luebke's-ochsenbein flap?	NTR-NR	2001 Apr	261
4. Indications for periapical surgery?	NTR-OR	2000 Apr	260
5. Flap designs for periapical surgery?	NTR-OR	1998 Oct	260
6. Flap design for endodontic surgeries?	NTR-NR	2001 Oct	260
7. Flap designs in surgical endodontics?	NTR-NR	2006 Apr	260

Brief notes

Question	University	Year	Page
1. Masseran kit?	NTR-NR	2002 Oct	232

28. Endodontic-Periodontic Interrelationship

Long essays

Short notes

Brief notes

29. Miscellaneous Topics

Long essays

Short notes

Question	University	Year	Page
1. MTA?	NTR-NR	2006 Oct	240
2. CMCP?	NTR-OR	1994 Nov	
	NTR-OR	1995 Oct	
3. Apical matrix?	NTR-NR	2005 Apr	
4. Cracked tooth syndrome?	NTR-OR	1991 Mar	163
5. Indications of optical surgery?	NTR-OR	1999 Apr	

Brief notes

Question	University	Year	Page
1. Masseran kit?	NTR-NR	2002 Oct	232
2. Treatment of open apex?	NTR-NR	2006 Oct	

PEDODONTICS

SYLLABUS

1. Introduction, definition, scope and importance of pedodontics.
2. Morphology of dentition and its applications—applied morphology and histology of deciduous and permanent teeth. Importance of first permanent molar.
3. Fundamentals of dental health.
4. Biological factors responsible for maintenance of dental and oral health.
5. Contributory local factors affecting oral health and plaque, etc.
6. Child psychology and management of child patient.
7. Examination, diagnosis and treatment planning.
8. Clinical pedodontics.
9. Setup of pedodontic clinic.
10. Teething disorders.
11. Developmental anomalies.
12. Dental caries in children with its prevention.
13. Restorative dentistry.
14. Pulp therapy and endodontics.
15. Space maintainers.
16. Treatment of traumatized teeth.
17. Management of problems of the primary and mixed dentition period.
18. Gingival and periodontal disorders in children and their management.
19. Stomatological conditions in children.
20. Management of handicapped children.
21. Mouth habits and their managements.
22. Dental materials in pedodontics.
23. Dental caries and its prevention.

SCHEME OF EXAMINATION

Theory

Theory – 70 Marks
Viva Voce – 10 Marks
Internal Assessment (Theory) – 20 Marks

Pedodontics (Part-A + Part-B / 35 + 35 = 70)

Subject	*Type of question*	*Marks offered*	*Total*
Part-A/Pedodontics	Long essays	9	1 x 9 = 09
	Short notes	4	4 x 4 = 16
	Brief notes	2	5 x 2 = 10
Part-B/Pedodontics	Long essays	9	1 x 9 = 09
	Short notes	4	4 x 4 = 16
	Brief notes	2	5 x 2 = 10

Clinicals

Clinicals – 70 Marks
Viva Voce – 10 Marks
Internal Assessment (Clinicals) – 20 Marks

REFERENCE BOOK

Pedodontics: Principle and Practice of Pedodontics – By Arthi Rao

AUTHOR ABBREVIATION

Arthi: Arthi Rao

Edition: 1st

QUESTION BANK ABBREVIATION

Question Bank

LE — Long essays
SN — Short notes
BN — Brief notes

University

NTRUHS — Nandamuri Taraka Rama Rao University of Health Sciences
NTRUHS-NR — NTRUHS–New Regulations
NTRUHS-OR — NTRUHS–Old Regulations

CONTENTS

Contd...

Contd...

Contd...

Contd...

Contd...

Contd...

PEDODONTICS

Arthi

1. Introduction to Pediatric Dentistry

Long essays

Short notes

1. Pedodontic triangle.	NTR-NR	1997 Apr	6
2. Define pediatric dentistry.	NTR-NR	2002 Apr	2
3. Pedodontic treatment triangle.	NTR-NR	2002 Apr	6
4. Definition and importance of pedodontics.	NTR-NR	2004 Apr	2

Brief notes

2. Case History and Examination

Long essays

1. Discuss case taking, clinical examination and diagnosis of trauma to anterior teeth.	NTR-NR	2006 Apr	15

Short notes

Brief notes

3. Diagnosis and Treatment Plan

Long essays

Short notes

Brief notes

4. Practice Management

Long essays

Short notes

1. Set-up of pedodontic clinic.	NTR-OR	1998 Apr	384

Brief notes

5. Child in Dental Office

Long essays

Short notes

Brief notes

6. Role of Dental Auxiliaries

Long essays

Short notes

1. Dental auxiliary.	NTR-NR	2000 Apr	380
2. Newzealand dental nurses.	NTR-OR	1997 Apr	381

Brief notes

7. Infection Control Procedures

Long essays

Short notes

Brief notes

8. Pediatric Radiology

Long essays

Short notes

1. Bite-wing radiographs.	NTR-NR	1998 Apr	291
	NTR-OR	1998 Oct	
2. Bite-wing radiographs in children.	NTR-NR	2002 Apr	291
	NTR-NR	2006 Apr	
3. Intraoral periapical radiography in children.	NTR-NR	2002 Oct	290

Brief notes

1. Bite-wing radiograph.	NTR-NR	2004 Oct	291

9. Theories of Child Development

Long essays

1. Describe the psychological development of child from birth to adolescent.	NTR-OR	1998 Oct	63
	NTR-NR	2005 Apr	
2. Discuss the role of learning theories in management of children in dental office.	NTR-NR	2006 Apr	65

Arthi

Short notes

1. Oedipus complex.	NTR-NR	2002 Apr	63
2. Oedipus conflict and Electra conflict.	NTR-NR	2004 Oct	63

Brief notes

1. Super ego.	NTR-NR	2006 Apr	62
2. Trust vs Mistrust.	NTR-NR	2002 Oct	

10. Emotional Development of Child

Long essays

1. Define and classify fear. Describe the methods for management of child in dental office.	NTR-NR	1999 Apr	68

Short notes

1. Fear.	NTR-NR	2004 Oct	68
2. Fear in pedodontia.	NTR-NR	1997 Oct	68
3. Define oral habit and fear.	NTR-OR	1992 Nov	68, 116

Brief notes

11. Parental Considerations of Child Behavior

Long essays

1. Describe the parental influences on the behavior of children during dental treatment.	NTR-OR	1992 Sep	74

Short notes

Brief notes

12. Behavioral Sciences and Its Applications

Long essays

1. How does dental office atmosphere affect behavior of the children?	NTR-NR	2002 Apr	
2. Discuss the causes of pain in children and write the methods and agents for controlling fear and pain in child dental patient.	NTR-NR	1998 Oct	83

Short notes

1. Wright's classification of behavior of children in dental office.	NTR-OR	2001 Oct	75

Brief notes

Arthi

13. Behavior Management

Long essays

	Question	University	Year	Page
1.	Enumerate the different types of child behavior and management techniques.	NTR-NR	2002 Apr	77
2.	Discuss various behavioral management of a 4 years old child throwing temper–tantrums.	NTR-NR	2001 Apr	77
3.	What is behavior management? How will you manage a fearful child or two years using a different behavior modification techniques?	NTR-NR	2000 Apr	77

Short notes

	Question	University	Year	Page
1.	TSD.	NTR-NR	1992 Nov	78
2.	TSD technique.	NTR-OR	1992 Apr	78
3.	HOME.	NTR-NR	1999 Nov	81
		NTR-NR	2004 Apr	
4.	HOME technique.	NTR-OR	1994 Apr	
5.	Handover month exercise (HOME).	NTR-NR	2001 Oct	81
		NTR-NR	2002 Oct	
6.	Modeling.	NTR-NR	1995 Apr	
		NTR-OR	1997 Apr	79
		NTR-OR	2000 Apr	
		NTR-NR	2004 Apr	
7.	Rewarding.	NTR-NR	1990 Feb	64, 70
8.	Restraining.	NTR-NR	2003 Apr	83
9.	Physical restrains.	NTR-NR	1997 Apr	82
10.	Aversive conditioning.	NTR-OR	1999 Oct	81
11.	Operant conditioning.	NTR-NR	2006 Oct	62

Brief notes

	Question	University	Year	Page
1.	Reinforcers.	NTR-NR	2006 Oct	79

14. Therapeutic Management

Long essays

	Question	University	Year	Page
1.	Classify pharmacological behavior management. Describe the effects, adverse effects, indications, and contraindications of Nitrous oxide analgesics.	NTR-NR	2000 Apr	83, 87

Short notes

	Question	University	Year	Page
1.	Conscious sedation in pediatric dentistry.	NTR-NR	1998 Apr	85

Brief notes

Arthi

15. Guidelines for Management of Handicapped Children

Long essays

1. Define handicap. Describe the management of handicapped child.	NTR-NR	1990 Feb	263

Short notes

1. Discuss various measures in the treatment and management of the handicapped children.	NTR-OR	1989 Feb	285

Brief notes

1. Definition of handicapped child.	NTR-NR	2006 Apr	263

16. Management of Medically Compromised Children

Long essays

1. Classify handicapped children. What precautions call your take while carrying out dental treatment for a patient suffering from hemophilia?	NTR-OR	1994 Apr	263
2. Define and classify the handicapped conditions in pedodontic patients and discuss the management of hemophilic child for an extraction of teeth.	NTR-OR	1995 Apr	263

Short notes

1. Measles.	NTR-OR	1992 Nov	344
	NTR-OR	1999 Apr	

Brief notes

17. Management of Children with Physically and Mentally Handicapped Children

Long essays

Short notes

1. Communicative disorders.	NTR-NR	2001 Oct	
2. Dental management of child with epilepsy.	NTR-NR	2006 Oct	279

Brief notes

18. Management of Children with Cleft Lip and Palate

Long essays

1. Classify cleft lip and left palates write briefly their pathogenesis, epidemiology, etiology and dental treatment.	NTR-NR	1998 Oct	

Short notes

1. Cleft palate. NTR-OR 1994 Apr
2. Ellis and Davey classification. NTR-NR 2006 Oct

Brief notes

19. Stages of Growth and Development (Prenatal)

Long essays

Short notes

Brief notes

20. Stages of Growth and Development (Postnatal)

Long essays

1. Describe the normal jaw structures of the newborn child and amount of calcified dentition in it. NTR-OR 1990 Feb 31

Short notes

Brief notes

21. Factors Affecting Growth

Long essays

Short notes

1. Hormones influencing growth. NTR-NR 2005 Apr 32

Brief notes

22. Growth Assessment

Long essays

Short notes

Brief notes

23. Growth Prediction and Visual Treatment Objectives

Long essays

Short notes

Brief notes

24. Eruption of Teeth

Long essays

Short notes

1. Teething.	NTR-NR	1994 Apr	50
	NTR-OR	1997 Oct	
	NTR-OR	1999 Oct	
	NTR-OR	2001 Oct	
2. Teething disorder.	NTR-OR	1999 Nov	50

Brief notes

25. Natal and Neonatal Teeth

Long essays

Short notes

1. Natal teeth.	NTR-NR	2003 Apr	51
2. Natal and neonatal teeth.	NTR-NR	1994 Nov	51
	NTR-OR	1997 Apr	
	NTR-OR	1998 Apr	

Brief notes

1. Natal and neonatal teeth.	NTR-NR	2006 Oct	51

26. Development of Occlusion

Long essays

1. Describe the development of occlusion from deciduous to permanent stages.	NTR-NR	2000 Apr	54

Short notes

1. Gum pads.	NTR-NR	2003 Apr	54
2. Primate space.	NTR-NR	1996 Apr	56
	NTR-OR	2001 Apr	
	NTR-NR	2001 Oct	
3. Leeway space.	NTR-NR	1998 Oct	58
	NTR-OR	2001 Apr	
4. Incisal liability.	NTR-OR	1989 Feb	58
	NTR-OR	1992 Apr	
	NTR-NR	2005 Apr	
5. Occlusion in deciduous dentition.	NTR-NR	1997 Oct	56
	NTR-OR	1998 Apr	
	NTR-OR	2001 Apr	
	NTR-NR	2004 Oct	

6. Importance of deciduous dentition.	NTR-NR	1997 Oct	47
7. Sequence of eruption of permanent teeth.	NTR-NR	1998 Oct	

Brief notes

1. Gum pads.	NTR-NR	2004 Oct	54
2. Incisal liability.	NTR-NR	2004 Oct	56
3. Primary molar occlusion.	NTR-NR	2006 Oct	56
4. Second primary molar relationship.	NTR-NR	2002 Oct	58

27. Self-correcting Anomalies

Long essays

Short notes

1. Ugly ducking stage.	NTR-NR	1996 Apr	59
	NTR-OR	1998 Apr	
	NTR-OR	1998 Oct	
	NTR-OR	1999 Apr	
	NTR-NR	2000 Apr	
	NTR-OR	2001 Apr	
	NTR-NR	2001 Oct	
	NTR-NR	2004 Oct	
2. Transient malocclusion.	NTR-NR	2006 Apr	60
3. Self-correcting anomalies.	NTR-OR	1998 Oct	60

Brief notes

28. Morphology of Deciduous Dentition

Long essays

Short notes

1. Mamelons.	NTR-NR	2003 Apr	
2. Importance of first permanent molar.	NTR-OR	1996 Apr	10
	NTR-NR	2002 Oct	
3. Applied morphology of primary and permanent molar teeth.	NTR-NR	2006 Apr	9
4. FDI system of counting of teeth.	NTR-OR	1989 Feb	

Brief notes

1. Mulberry molars.	NTR-NR	2006 Oct	

29. Disturbances of Teeth and Surrounding Structures

Long essays

Short notes

1. Mesiodens.	NTR-NR	2001 Oct	332
	NTR-NR	2003 Apr	
2. Twinning.	NTR-NR	2005 Apr	331
3. Talon's cap.	NTR-NR	2005 Apr	
4. Submerged teeth.	NTR-OR	1998 Oct	
	NTR-NR	2001 Oct	
5. Enamel hypoplasia.	NTR-OR	2001 Apr	335
6. Turner's hypoplasia.	NTR-OR	1990 Feb	336
7. Gemination and fusion.	NTR-NR	2004 Apr	332
	NTR-NR	2006 Apr	
8. Amelogenesis imperfecta.	NTR-NR	1998 Oct	336
9. Anomalies of the number of teeth.	NTR-NR	2006 Oct	332

Brief notes

1. Mesiodens.	NTR-NR	2003 Apr	333
2. Turner's hypoplasia.	NTR-NR	2003 Apr	336
	NTR-NR	2006 Oct	

30. Regressive Alternations of Teeth

Long essays

Short notes

Brief notes

31. Pulp and Periapical Diseases

Long essays

Short notes

1. Pink tooth.	NTR-NR	2003 Apr	252
2. Dentoalveolar abscess.	NTR-NR	2003 Apr	

Brief notes

32. Gingival and Periodontal Diseases

Long essays

1. Classify periodontal diseases in children and adolescents. Discuss localized aggressive periodontitis.	NTR-NR	2003 Apr	308

Short notes

1.	ANUG.	NTR-OR	2001 Oct	309
2.	Herpetic gingivitis.	NTR-OR	1999 Oct	308
3.	Vincent's infection.	NTR-OR	1995 Apr	309
4.	Scorbutic gingivitis.	NTR-OR	1996 Apr	310
5.	Gingival recession.	NTR-NR	1992 Nov	
6.	Gingival enlargements.	NTR-NR	2004 Apr	307
7.	Periodontium in children.	NTR-OR	1999 Oct	306
8.	Juvenile periodontitis.	NTR-OR	1997 Oct	310
		NTR-OR	1998 Apr	
9.	Acute herpetic gingivostomatitis.	NTR-NR	2000 Apr	308
10.	Acute necrotizing ulcerative gingivitis.	NTR-NR	2006 Apr	309
11.	General principles of treatment of periodontal conditions in children.	NTR-NR	1998 Oct	

Brief notes

1.	Fenestration.	NTR-NR	2005 Apr	309
2.	Dilantin sodium.	NTR-NR	2005 Apr	
3.	Eruption gingivitis.	NTR-NR	2003 Apr	308
		NTR-NR	2005 Apr	
4.	Clinical features of juvenile periodontitis.	NTR-NR	2005 Apr	310

33. TMJ Disorders in Children

Long essays

Short notes

Brief notes

34. Acquired Mucoskeletal Disorders

Long essays

Short notes

Brief notes

35. Acquired Salivary Gland Disorders

Long essays

Short notes

Brief notes

Arthi

36. Commonly Seen Cysts and Tumors in Children

Long essays

Short notes

1. Bhon's nodules.	NTR-OR	1992 Apr	52

Brief notes

37. Congenital Abnormalities in Children

Long essays

Short notes

1. Erythroblastosis fetalis.	NTR-NR	1998 Oct	

Brief notes

38. Chromosomal Abnormalities in Children

Long essays

Short notes

1. Autism.	NTR-OR	1996 Apr	281

Brief notes

39. Commonly Seen Syndromes in Children

Long essays

Short notes

1. Trisomy.	NTR-OR	2001 Oct	359
2. AIDS in children.	NTR-NR	1998 Oct	345
3. Down's syndrome.	NTR-OR	1998 Oct	358
	NTR-OR	1999 Oct	
	NTR-NR	2004 Apr	

Brief notes

40. Pernicious Oral Habits

Long essays

1. Define and classify oral habits. Describe the management of mouthbreathing and thumb-sucking.	NTR-OR	1999 Apr	116

Short notes

1. Mouthbreathing.	NTR-NR	1990 Feb	117
	NTR-OR	1995 Apr	
	NTR-OR	1998 Apr	
	NTR-OR	1998 Aug	
	NTR-OR	2001 Oct	
	NTR-NR	2003 Apr	
2. Tongue thrusting.	NTR-NR	1998 Apr	120
3. Masochistic habits.	NTR-NR	2000 Apr	126
4. Thumbsucking habits.	NTR-OR	1997 Apr	117
	NTR-OR	2001 Apr	
5. Define oral habit diagnosis fear.	NTR-NR	1992 Nov	116

Brief notes

1. Thumbsucking.	NTR-NR	2004 Oct	117
2. Vestibular screen.	NTR-NR	2005 Apr	123

41. Development of Malocclusion

Long essays

Short notes

1. Crossbite in anterior teeth.	NTR-NR	2006 Apr	97
2. Normal forces of occlusion.	NTR-OR	1998 Apr	

Brief notes

42. Model Analysis in Primary Dentition

Long essays

Short notes

Brief notes

43. Diagnosis and Management of Malocclusion

Long essays

Short notes

1. Tongue blade therapy.	NTR-NR	1992 Nov	97
	NTR-OR	1997 Apr	

Brief notes

1. Tongue blade therapy.	NTR-NR	2005 Apr	97
	NTR-NR	2006 Oct	
2. Correction of anterior crossbite.	NTR-NR	2004 Apr	97

Arthi

44. Preventive and Interceptive Orthodontics

Long essays

1. Discuss recent concepts on interceptive orthodontics for children.	NTR-NR	2006 Oct	96
2. What are the indications for space maintainers and describe the various types of the some?	NTR-NR	1998 Apr	104
3. Define and classify space maintainers write in detail about distal shoespace maintainers.	NTR-NR	2004 Oct	103
4. Define and classify space maintainers and describe the Willet's guiding space maintainer.	NTR-OR	1999 Nov	103
5. Define and classify space maintainers. What factors would you consider before giving space maintainer to the child patient?	NTR-OR	1989 Feb	103
6. Define serial extraction. Discuss the indication, contraindication and the procedure of serial extraction.	NTR-NR	2001 Oct	

Short notes

1. Space management.	NTR-NR	1999 Apr	103
2. Space regainer.	NTR-NR	2004 Apr	111
3. Steri space regainer.	NTR-NR	1998 Oct	
	NTR-NR	2001 Oct	
4. Space maintainers.	NTR-OR	1990 Aug	103
5. Nance's appliance.	NTR-OR	1994 Apr	109
	NTR-NR	2004 Apr	
6. Distal shoe space maintainer.	NTR-NR	1992 Apr	110
	NTR-OR	1998 Apr	
	NTR-OR	2000 Apr	
	NTR-OR	2001 Apr	
	NTR-OR	2001 Oct	
7. Removable space maintainer.	NTR-NR	2006 Oct	104
8. Band and loop space maintainer.	NTR-NR	2002 Oct	106
9. Indications of serial extraction.	NTR-NR	2005 Apr	

Brief notes

45. Etiology of Dental Caries

Long essays

Short notes

1. Arrested caries.	NTR-OR	1994 Apr	140
2. Zones of dental caries in enamel and dentin.	NTR-NR	2006 Apr	138

Brief notes

1. Hidden caries.	NTR-NR	2005 Oct	
2. Stephen's curve.	NTR-NR	2005 Oct	137

46. Diet and Dental Caries

Long essays

Short notes

1. Trace elements.	NTR-NR	1998 Oct	136
2. Diet and dental caries.	NTR-NR	2006 Apr	133
3. Diet factor in dental caries.	NTR-NR	2001 Oct	133
4. Cariogenic diet and substitutes.	NTR-OR	1992 Apr	133

Brief notes

1. Cariostatic trace elements.	NTR-NR	2005 Apr	136

47. Early Childhood Caries

Long essays

1. Define rampart caries, write in detail about it.	NTR-NR	2001 Oct	141
2. Define rampart caries. How will you manage the same?	NTR-NR	1998 Oct	141
3. Define rampart caries. Discuss its etiology, clinical features and management.	NTR-NR NTR-NR	2004 Apr 2005 Apr	141
4. Define rampart caries. Discuss the etiology, clinical features and step by step management of the same.	NTR-NR	2002 Oct	141
5. Classify dental caries. Give a detailed description of how will you treat a case of nursing bottle caries?	NTR-OR	1996 Apr	141
6. Define rampant caries. How would you differentiate rampant caries from nursing bottle carrier? Discuss in detail management of a case of rampart caries.	NTR-NR	1998 Apr	141

Short notes

1. Nursing caries.	NTR-OR	1999 Oct	142
2. Nursing bottle caries.	NTR-NR	1998 Apr	142
3. Define rampart caries.	NTR-NR	2002 Apr	141
4. Baby bottle syndrome.	NTR-NR	2000 Apr	142

Brief notes

48. Infants and Oral Health

Long essays

	Question			
1.	Describe the various biological factors responsible for the maintenance of oral health.	NTR-OR	1992 Nov	

Short notes

Brief notes

49. Saliva and Oral Health

Long essays

Short notes

Brief notes

50. Plaque and Oral Health

Long essays

	Question			
1.	Define dentifrice. Give composition of the same. Discuss the mechanical and chemical methods of plaque control.	NTR-OR	1999 Oct	198

Short notes

	Question			
1.	Dental plaque.	NTR-OR	2001 Oct	130
2.	Disclosing solution.	NTR-NR	2000 Apr	199
3.	Role of toothbrushes.	NTR-OR	2000 Apr	
4.	Anti-plaque mouth rinses.	NTR-NR	2004 Apr	
5.	Self-control of plaque.	NTR-NR	2004 Oct	
6.	Chemical control of dental plaques.	NTR-OR	1992 Apr	199
7.	Brushing and flossing for children.	NTR-NR	2006 Oct	196
8.	Brushing methods for children.	NTR-OR	2001 Oct	196
9.	Fones method of toothbrushing.	NTR-NR	1998 Oct	196
10.	Toothbrushing techniques in children.	NTR-NR	1998 Apr	196
11.	Modification of toothbrush for handicapped children.	NTR-OR	1992 Apr	

Brief notes

	Question			
1.	Dental floss.	NTR-NR	2003 Apr	199
2.	Plaque control.	NTR-OR	1990 Feb	

51. Home Oral Hygiene Care

Long essays

Short notes

Brief notes

52. Nutritional Considerations for Children

Long essays

Short notes

Brief notes

53. Counseling of the Child

Long essays

Short notes

1. Parent counseling. NTR-NR 1998 Apr 197

Brief notes

54. Diet Counseling

Long essays

Short notes

Brief notes

55. Genetic Counseling

Long essays

Short notes

Brief notes

56. Diagnosis of Dental Caries

Long essays

Short notes

Brief notes

57. Caries Activity Tests

Long essays

Short notes

1. Snyder's test. NTR-NR 1992 Nov 182
   NTR-OR 1998 Nov

2. Caries activity tests. NTR-OR 1994 Apr 181
NTR-OR 1997 Oct
NTR-OR 2000 Apr
3. Caries susceptibility tests. NTR-NR 1999 Apr 181

Brief notes

58. Caries Vaccine

Long essays

Short notes

1. Caries vaccines. NTR-NR 1998 Apr
NTR-OR 1998 Oct

Brief notes

59. Pit and Fissure Sealant

Long essays

1. What are fissure sealants? Enumerate in detail their importance indications, contraindications and their method of application. NTR-NR 2000 Apr 188

Short notes

1. Fissure sealants. NTR-NR 1998 Apr 188
2. Pit and fissure sealants. NTR-NR 1996 Apr 188
NTR-OR 1999 Apr
NTR-OR 1998 Oct
NTR-OR 1999 Oct
NTR-NR 2005 Apr
3. Preventive resin restorations. NTR-NR 2006 Apr 187

Brief notes

60. Atraumatic Restorative Treatment

Long essays

Short notes

1. Prophylactic odontotomy. NTR-OR 1997 Oct 187
2. Hyatt prophylactic odontotomy. NTR-OR 1992 Nov 187

Brief notes

1. Atraumatic restorative treatment. NTR-NR 2005 Apr 186

Arthi

61. Fluorides and Dental Health

Long essays

1. Give a detailed account of role of fluorides in preventive dentistry.	NTR-NR	1998 Apr	210
2. Define water fluoridation. Discuss its feasibility in India.	NTR-NR	2004 Apr	208
3. Define fluoridation. Discuss suitable method of systemic fluoridation for Indian population.	NTR-OR	2001 Oct	208
4. Describe the role of topical fluorides in the prevention of dental caries.	NTR-NR	1997 Apr	210
5. Describe the role of systemic fluorides in the prevention of dental caries.	NTR-NR	1996 Apr	208
6. Discuss the importance of systemic fluorides in prevention of tooth decay, state the mechanism of its action in short.	NTR-NR	1990 Apr	208
7. Discuss in detail the role of fluoride varnish used for the prevention of dental caries.	NTR-OR	1992 Nov	214
8. Define water fluoridation. Describe the various systemic methods for the prevention of dental caries.	NTR-OR	1990 Aug	208

Short notes

1. APF gel.	NTR-NR	1999 Feb	211
	NTR-OR	1995 Apr	
	NTR-OR	1997 Apr	
	NTR-OR	1998 Apr	
	NTR-OR	1999 Apr	
	NTR-NR	2000 Apr	
2. Fluoride gels.	NTR-NR	1999 Oct	212
3. Fluoride varnish.	NTR-NR	2000 Apr	214
	NTR-NR	2002 Oct	
4. Fluoride month wash.	NTR-OR	2001 Apr	213
5. Brudevold solution.	NTR-NR	1992 Nov	
6. Stannous fluoride.	NTR-OR	1999 Oct	211
7. Knutson's technique.	NTR-NR	1997 Oct	211
	NTR-NR	2001 Oct	
8. Water fluoridation.	NTR-OR	1989 Feb	208
9. Milk fluoridation.	NTR-OR	1998 Apr	210
10. School water fluoridation.	NTR-NR	1999 Oct	209
11. Defluoridators.	NTR-NR	1998 Oct	217
12. Nalgonda technique.	NTR-OR	1997 Oct	218
13. Topical fluorides.	NTR-OR	1999 Apr	210
14. Shoe leather survey.	NTR-NR	2004 Oct	207

15. Chocking phenomenon.	NTR-NR	2004 Apr	211
16. Mechanism of action of fluoride in preventing dental caries.	NTR-NR	2000 Apr	207

Brief notes

1. Brudevold solution.	NTR-NR	2005 Apr	212

62. Pediatric Restorative Materials

Long essays

Short notes

1. Willey's inlay.	NTR-NR	1990 Aug	
	NTR-OR	1992 Nov	
2. Cavity liners.	NTR-OR	1995 Apr	
3. Glutaraldehyde.	NTR-OR	2001 Apr	229
4. Calcium hydroxide.	NTR-NR	1998 Apr	224
	NTR-NR	2000 Apr	
5. High copper alloys.	NTR-OR	1992 Apr	
	NTR-OR	2000 Apr	
6. Dentin bonding agents.	NTR-OR	2001 Apr	167
7. Zinc phosphate cement.	NTR-OR	1999 Apr	
8. Glass ionomer cements.	NTR-NR	1994 Apr	
	NTR-OR	1997 Oct	155
	NTR-OR	1998 Oct	
	NTR-OR	2001 Apr	
	NTR-NR	2003 Apr	
9. Use of glass ionomer in pediatric dentistry.	NTR-NR	2001 Oct	158

Brief notes

1. Cavity varnish.	NTR-NR	2003 Apr	

63. Principles and Concepts of Cavity Preparation

Long essays

Short notes

1. Tunnel preparation.	NTR-NR	2002 Apr	149
2. Class II cavity restoration (Amalgam) is a failure – Discuss.	NTR-NR	1990 Feb	148
3. Modification of cavity preparation in primary molar for class II restoration.	NTR-OR	2001 Oct	149

Brief notes

1. Proximal slicing of primary teeth.	NTR-NR	2006 Apr	149

Arthi

64. Matrices, Retainers and Wedges

Long essays

Short notes

1. Separators.	NTR-NR	2000 Apr	149
2. Matrices used in pedodontics.	NTR-OR	1992 Nov	149
3. Matrices used in pediatric dentistry.	NTR-OR	1998 Oct	149

Brief notes

65. Rubber Dam Application in Pediatric Dentistry

Long essays

Short notes

1. Isolation.	NTR-NR	1999 Apr	150
2. Rubber dam in pedodontics.	NTR-NR	2001 Oct	151

Brief notes

66. Restoration of Primary Carious Teeth

Long essays

1. Discuss the various procedures in the management of deep canine lesions in primary and young permanent molars.	NTR-OR	1992 Apr	
2. Describe the management of deep carious lesions of tooth No 46 in a seven-year-old child.	NTR-NR	2006 Oct	
3. Class II amalgam restoration is a failure in primary second molar. Discuss.	NTR-OR	1997 Apr	

Short notes

Brief notes

67. Crowns in Pediatric Dentistry

Long essays

Short notes

1. Stainless steel crown.	NTR-OR	1990 Aug	170
	NTR-OR	1995 Apr	
	NTR-OR	1997 Apr	
	NTR-NR	2000 Apr	
	NTR-NR	2003 Apr	
	NTR-NR	2004 Oct	

2. Polycarbonate crowns. NTR-NR 1992 Apr; NTR-OR 1996 Apr; NTR-OR 2001 Apr

Brief notes

68. Objectives and Diagnostic Procedures

Long essays

Short notes

Brief notes

69. Endodontic Treatment Modalities

Long essays

1. What is the difference between apexogensis and apexification? Explain in detail. NTR-NR 2003 Apr 232
2. Define pulpotomy. Describe the procedure of pulpotomy of second mandibular primary molar. NTR-NR 2001 Oct 227
3. Define pulpotomy. Describe the technique and pulpal tissue changes following formocresol pulpotomy in primary molar. NTR-NR 2001 Oct 228
4. Describe the procedure in treating a young permanent fractured central incisor with wide apical foramen and necrotic pulp. NTR-OR 1989 Feb
5. Define pulpotomy. Give the indications and contraindication. Describe the histological picture of dental pulp after a glutaraldehyde pulpotomy. Why is glutaraldehyde preferred over formocresol, for the same? NTR-OR 1999 Oct 227
6. A child of 6 years has an abscess associated with lower left first deciduous molar, which is nonvital. The second deciduous molar on the same side has a vital carious exposure. Discuss your line of treatment. NTR-OR 1997 Oct

Short notes

1. Apexification. NTR-NR 1992 Apr 232; NTR-OR 1996 Apr; NTR-OR 1997 Oct; NTR-OR 1998 Oct; NTR-OR 2000 Apr; NTR-NR 2000 Apr; NTR-NR 2001 Oct

2. Glutaraldehyde.	NTR-NR	2001 Apr	229
3. Direct pulp capping.	NTR-NR	2000 Apr	225
4. Indirect pulp capping.	NTR-NR	1998 Oct	224
5. Pulp capping agents.	NTR-OR	1999 Apr	225
	NTR-OR	1999 Oct	
	NTR-OR	2000 Apr	
	NTR-NR	2004 Apr	
	NTR-NR	2006 Apr	
6. Pulp vitality tests.	NTR-NR	2003 Apr	223
7. Lasers in pulpotomy.	NTR-NR	2002 Oct	228
8. Formocresol pulpotomy.	NTR-NR	2004 Oct	228
9. Pulpotomy medicaments.	NTR-NR	1998 Apr	
10. Sweet formocresol pulpotomy.	NTR-OR	1997 Apr	228
11. Electrosurgical pulpotomy.	NTR-NR	2003 Apr	231
12. Root canal filling materials used in 75.	NTR-NR	1992 Nov	
13. Obturating materials for primary teeth.	NTR-NR	2005 Apr	231

Brief notes

1. Formocresol.	NTR-NR	2006 Oct	228
2. Indirect pulp capping.	NTR-NR	2004 Apr	224

70. Traumatic Injuries of Teeth and Management

Long essays

1. Give detailed account of reactions of dental pulp to traumatic injury.	NTR-OR	1994 Apr	245
2. Classify the injuries to anterior teeth (any one classification) and discuss in detail the management of traumatized permanent central incisor a 7 years old child with pulpal involvement.	NTR-OR	2001 Apr	235
3. A 9-year-old child sustained fracture of upper right central incisor the fracture-involved enamel and dentine but without pulp exposure. Discuss yours immediate, intermediate and permanent treatment in the patient.	NTR-OR	1998 Apr	243

Short notes

1. Splints.	NTR-OR	1994 Apr	251
	NTR-NR	1998 Apr	
2. Ellis classification of fracture of anterior teeth.	NTR-NR	1998 Oct	238
3. Classify traumatic injuries to anterior teeth (Ellis classification).	NTR-NR	2002 Apr	238

Brief notes

1. Intrusive luxation.	NTR-NR	2006 Apr	242
2. Ellis class 5 injuries.	NTR-NR	2006 Oct	235

71. Sports Related Dental Injuries

Long essays

Short notes

Brief notes

1. Non-accidental injury.	NTR-NR	2006 Apr	

72. Mouth Guards

Long essays

Short notes

1. Oral guards.	NTR-NR	1998 Oct	
2. Mouth guards.	NTR-NR	1996 Apr	255
	NTR-NR	2001 Oct	
3. Mouth protectors.	NTR-NR	1999 Apr	
4. Mouth protections.	NTR-OR	1992 Apr	255
	NTR-OR	1994 Nov	255

Brief notes

73. Principles of Pediatric Pharmacology

Long essays

Short notes

1. Premedication in children.	NTR-OR	1989 Feb	83
	NTR-OR	1995 Apr	
2. Premedication in pedodontics.	NTR-OR	2001 Oct	83
3. Drug dosage calculations for children.	NTR-OR	2001 Oct	85

Brief notes

1. Young's rule.	NTR-NR	2006 Apr	85
2. Premedication.	NTR-NR	2006 Oct	83

74. Analgesics and Antimicrobial Drugs

Long essays

Short notes

1. Amoxicillin.	NTR-NR	2000 Apr	
2. Pigmentation in tetracycline therapy.	NTR-NR	1998 Apr	347

Brief notes

1. Clotrimazole.	NTR-NR	2006 Oct	

75. Local Anesthesia and General Anesthesia

Long essays

Short notes

Brief notes

1. Composition of local anesthetic solution.	NTR-NR	2002 Oct	297

76. Conscious Sedation

Long essays

Short notes

1. Diazepam.	NTR-OR	1999 Oct	90
2. Conscious sedation in pediatric dentistry.	NTR-NR	1998 Apr	85

Brief notes

77. Vaccination for Children

Long essays

Short notes

1. Immunization in dentistry.	NTR-OR	1999 Nov	

Brief notes

78. Nerve Blocks

Long essays

Short notes

1. Mandibular block in children.	NTR-NR	2002 Apr	295
2. Inferior alveolar nerve block in a 5 years old children.	NTR-NR	2005 Apr	295

Brief notes

79. Extractions in Pediatric Dentistry

Long essays

Short notes

1. Premature extraction of deciduous teeth.	NTR-OR	1989 Feb	

Brief notes

80. Minor Oral Surgery in Pediatric Dentistry

Long essays

Short notes

Brief notes

81. Pediatric Medical Emergencies

Long essays

Short notes

Brief notes

82. Pediatric Prosthodontics

Long essays

Short notes

Brief notes

83. Latest Advances in Genetics

Long essays

Short notes

Brief notes

84. Child Abuse and Neglect

Long essays

Short notes

1. Child abuse.	NTR-NR	1997 Oct	257
	NTR-OR	1998 Apr	
2. Orofacial signs of sexual abuse.	NTR-OR	1997 Oct	257

Brief notes

85. Bitemarks

Long essays

Short notes

Brief notes

86. Dental Age Assessment

Long essays

Short notes

Brief notes

87. General Epidemiology

Long essays

Short notes

1. Cohort study. NTR-OR 1995 Apr

Brief notes

88. Principles of Biostatistics

Long essays

Short notes

1. Normal curve. NTR-OR 1995 Apr
   NTR-NR 2005 Apr
2. Measurements of central tendency. NTR-NR 2002 Apr

Brief notes

89. Indices Used in Pediatric Dentistry

Long essays

1. Define index. Describe step by step procedure of assessing dental caries status of school children of Hyderabad city. NTR-OR 1998 Apr 373

Short notes

1. Caries indices. NTR-OR 1990 Aug 375
2. Caries index for primary dentition. NTR-NR 2002 Oct 376

Brief notes

90. Miscellaneous Topics

Long essays

1.	Compare the differences in the spread of carious lesions in deciduous and permanent teeth and its influence on cavity preparation on these teeth.	NTR-OR	1989 Feb

Short notes

1.	Caridex.	NTR-OR	1994 Apr
2.	Keye's triad.	NTR-OR	2001 Apr
3.	Staining of teeth.	NTR-OR	2000 Apr
4.	Thixotrophic gel.	NTR-NR	2003 Apr
5.	Audio-visual aids.	NTR-NR	2005 Apr
6.	Pre-cooperative children.	NTR-NR	2002 Oct
7.	Tooth numbering system.	NTR-OR	1999 Oct
8.	Battered child syndrome.	NTR-OR	1996 Apr
9.	Nerve supply of tooth No 26 (FDI).	NTR-NR	2003 Apr
10.	Specific effects of premature tooth loss.	NTR-NR	1998 Oct

Brief notes

1.	Ataxia.	NTR-NR	2006 Apr
2.	Subpoena.	NTR-NR	1997 Apr

ORTHODONTICS

SYLLABUS

1. Definition, aims, objectives and scope of orthodontics
2. Growth and development of jaws, teeth, face an skull and establishment of normal occlusion
3. Genetics as applied to orthodontics
4. Normal occlusion and its characteristics. Factors responsible for establishment and maintained of normal occlusion
5. Malocclusion—types and different classifications
6. History taking and examination of patient and case analysis and differential diagnosis including cephalometrics and treatment planning
7. Preventive and interceptive treatment of malocclusion
8. Extractions in orthodontics
9. Appliances used in orthodontic treatment—adequate knowledge of removable appliances, mechanical appliances and functional appliances, elementary knowledge of fixed appliances
10. Tissue changes incident to orthodontic treatment
11. Retention after treatment and relapse
12. Materials used in orthodontics
13. Habit breaking appliances

SCHEME OF EXAMINATION

Theory

Theory	–	70 Marks
Viva Voce	–	10 Marks
Internal Assessment (Theory)	–	20 Marks

Orthodontics (Part-A + Part-B / 35 + 35 = 70)

Subject	*Type of question*	*Marks offered*	*Total*
Part-A/Orthodontics	Long essays	9	1 x 9 = 09
	Short notes	4	4 x 4 = 16
	Brief notes	2	5 x 2 = 10
Part-B/Orthodontics	Long essays	9	1 x 9 = 09
	Short notes	4	4 x 4 = 16
	Brief notes	2	5 x 2 = 10

Clinicals

Clinicals	–	70 Marks
Viva Voce	–	10 Marks
Internal Assessment (Clinicals)	–	20 Marks

REFERENCE BOOK

Orthodontics: The Art and Science of Orthodontics – By SI Bhalaji

AUTHOR ABBREVIATION

Bhalaji: SI Bhalaji

Edition: 3rd

QUESTION BANK ABBREVIATION

Question Bank

LE — Long essays
SN — Short notes
BN — Brief notes

University

NTRUHS — Nandamuri Taraka Rama Rao University of Health Sciences
NTRUHS-NR — NTRUHS–New Regulations
NTRUHS-OR — NTRUHS–Old Regulations

CONTENTS

Contd...

Contd...

ORTHODONTICS

Bhalaji

1. Introduction to Orthodontics

Long essays

1. Define orthodontics. Describe about aims and science of orthodontics.	NTR-NR	1998 Apr	12

Short notes

1. Jackson's triad.	NTR-NR	2001 Oct	3
2. Aims of orthodontics.	NTR-NR	2001 Oct	2
3. Aims and objectives of orthodontics.	NTR-NR	2004 Oct	2

Brief notes

1. Definition and scope of orthodontics.	NTR-NR	2004 Apr	3, 4

2. General Principles and Concepts

Long essays

1. Define growth and development. Mention the various theories of growth and write in detail functional matrix hypothesis?	NTR-OR	1995 Oct	7

Short notes

1. Growth spurts	NTR-NR	1991 Mar	9
	NTR-OR	1994 Nov	
	NTR-OR	1997 Apr	
	NTR-OR	1998 Apr	
	NTR-OR	1998 Oct	
	NTR-NR	2003 Oct	
2. Growth sites	NTR-NR	2002 Apr	
3. Growth curve	NTR-NR	1999 Apr	
4. Pre-pubertal growth spurt	NTR-NR	2005 Oct	9
5. Pre-pubertal growth periods	NTR-OR	2000 Apr	9
6. Functional matrix theory	NTR-OR	1997 May	16

Brief notes

1. Growth spurts	NTR-NR	2003 Apr	9
	NTR-NR	2006 Oct	
2. Twin studies	NTR-NR	2006 Oct	489

3. Growth and Development of Cranial and Facial Structures

Long essays

Question	University	Year	Page
1. Describe in detail prenatal and post-natal growth of mandible.	NTR-NR	1997 Oct	21
	NTR-OR	2001 Oct	
2. Prenatal and post-natural growth and development of maxilla explain in detail.	NTR-NR	1993 May	24
3. Discuss prenatal and postnatal growth of mandible and its clinical application in orthodontics?	NTR-NR	2005 Apr	21
4. Discuss pre-natal and postnatal growth of mandible and its clinical implications in orthodontics?	NTR-NR	2006 Oct	21
5. Define growth and development. What are the theories of growth? How growth disturbances can cause malocclusion?	NTR-NR	2006 Apr	16

Short notes

Question	University	Year	Page
1. Synchondrosis	NTR-NR	1999 Apr	80
		2002 Oct	
2. Mechanism of bone growth	NTR-NR	2006 Aug	

Brief notes

Question	University	Year	Page
1. Sutural growth	NTR-NR	2001 Apr	31

4. Development of Dentition and Occlusion

Long essays

Question	University	Year	Page
1. Describe the development of normal occlusion?	NTR-OR	1990 Jul	39
2. Discuss the various stages of development of occlusion from birth to adolescent?	NTR-NR	2004 Oct	39

Short notes

Question	University	Year	Page
1. Gum pads	NTR-NR	1993 Oct	40
	NTR-NR	2004 Apr	
2. Primate spaces	NTR-NR	2003 Apr	41
	NTR-NR	2005 Apr	
3. Incisal liability	NTR-NR	2000 Apr	44
	NTR-NR	2004 Oct	
4. Ugly ducking stage	NTR-NR	1992 Nov	48
	NTR-OR	1994 Nov	
	NTR-OR	2001 Apr	
	NTR-NR	2004 Oct	
5. Free way space	NTR-NR	1999 Apr	128
6. Leeway space	NTR-OR	1999 Apr	44

			Bhalaji
7. Leeway space of Nance	NTR-NR	1993 Oct	44
	NTR-NR	2004 Oct	
	NTR-NR	2006 Apr	
8. Distal flush terminal plans	NTR-NR	1995 Oct	
9. Flush terminal plane	NTR-OR	1997 May	
10. Theories of eruption	NTR-NR	2006 Apr	182
11. Sequence of eruption of permanent teeth?	NTR-OR	1997 May	45

Brief notes

1. Primate spacing	NTR-NR	2002 Oct	41
	NTR-NR	2005 Apr	
2. Incisal liability	NTR-NR	2003 Apr	44
	NTR-NR	2005 Apr	
	NTR-NR	2006 Oct	
3. Flush terminal plane	NTR-NR	2004 Oct	
4. Stages of eruption of permanent teeth	NTR-NR	2006 Oct	45

5. Functional Development

Long essays

Short notes

1. Trajectories of occlusal forces	NTR-NR	2005 Apr	53
2. Trajectories of force in mandible	NTR-NR	1993 May	54
3. Wolf's law of transformations of bone	NTR-NR	1992 Nov	54

Brief notes

1. Trajectories	NTR-NR	2004 Oct	53
2. Wolfe's law	NTR-NR	2005 Apr	59

6. Occlusion—Basic Concepts

Long essays

1. What are six keys of normal occlusion? State how Ackerman profit system is an improvement over Angle's classification?	NTR-NR	2000 Apr	59

Short notes

1. Curse of Spee	NTR-NR	1999 Apr	56
2. Overjet and overbite	NTR-OR	1994 Nov	127
3. Occlusion and malocclusion	NTR-OR	1990 Feb	55
4. Normal occlusion concept	NTR-OR	1993 May	53

Brief notes

7. Classification of Malocclusion

Long essays

Question	Board	Year	Page
1. What is classification? Discuss the different classification on malocclusion. What is the latest classification on malocclusion?	NTR-NR	2001 Apr	1
2. Define various classifications of malocclusion and explain in detail Angle's classification and validity of Angle's classification?	NTR-OR	1994 Nov	66, 69
3. Describe the Angle's classification of malocclusion and mention the limitations of this classification?	NTR-OR	1990 Jul	69, 75
4. What are six keys of normal occlusion? State how Ackerman profit system is an improvement over Angle's classification.	NTR-NR	2000 Apr	59, 79

Short notes

Question	Board	Year	Page
1. Bennett classification.	NTR-NR	1993 Oct	78
2. Simon's classification of malocclusion.	NTR-NR	1998 Apr	77
	NTR-NR	2001 Oct	
3. Validity of angle's classification.	NTR-NR	1997 Oct	
	NTR-NR	2005 Oct	
4. Draw backs of Angle's classification.	NTR-NR	1999 Oct	75
	NTR-NR	2002 Apr	
5. Pseudo class III malocclusion.	NTR-NR	1992 Nov	75
	NTR-NR	2002 Oct	
	NTR-NR	2004 Apr	
6. Clinical features of class III malocclusion.	NTR-NR	1998 Apr	75
7. Clinical features of Class II div 2.	NTR-OR	2001 Apr	74
	NTR-NR	2002 Apr	

Brief notes

Question	Board	Year	Page
1. F-H plane.	NTR-NR	2005 Apr	148
2. Simon's classification.	NTR-NR	2006 Apr	77
3. Frankfort Horizontal plane.	NTR-NR	2004 Apr	148

8. Etiology of Malocclusion

Long essays

Question	Board	Year	Page
1. Define malocclusions? Discuss etiology of malocclusion.	NTR-NR	1999 Apr	82
2. Explain in detail, etiology of malocclusion.	NTR-OR	1997 May	82
3. Discuss the local causes of malocclusion.	NTR-NR	2002 Oct	82
4. Discuss the general causes for malocclusion.	NTR-NR	2002 Apr	82

			Bhalaji

Short notes

1. Teratogens.	NTR-NR	1999 Apr	440
2. Factors causing malocclusion.	NTR-OR	1989 Jul	82
3. Post-natal causes for malocclusion.	NTR-NR	2002 Apr	82
4. Local factors causing malocclusion.	NTR-OR	1993 Oct	82
5. Local factors in etiology of malocclusion.	NTR-NR	1998 Apr	82

Brief notes

1. Dilacerated tooth.	NTR-NR	2004 Apr	90
2. Submerged tooth.	NTR-NR	2004 Apr	94
3. Supplemental teeth.	NTR-NR	2006 Apr	85

9. Oral Habits

Long essays

1. Discuss the role of lip and tongue in relation to normal occlusion.	NTR-OR	1990 Feb	98
2. Enumerate the etiological factors causing mouth breathing and tongue thrust in children and discuss the line of treatment.	NTR-NR	2003 Apr	104
3. Define malocclusion. Classify etiology of malocclusion. Discuss clinical pictures and management of thumbsucking habit.	NTR-NR	2005 Oct	97

Short notes

1. Mouthbreathing.	NTR-NR	1999 Apr	104
	NTR-OR	2001 Oct	
2. Thumbsucking habit.	NTR-NR	1990 Jul	97
	NTR-OR	1992 Nov	
	NTR-OR	1997 May	
	NTR-OR	1998 Oct	
	NTR-NR	2004 Oct	
3. Sucking and suckling.	NTR-NR	2000 Apr	97
4. Tongue thrusting habit.	NTR-NR	1993 May	107
	NTR-OR	1995 Oct	
	NTR-OR	1997 Oct	
	NTR-NR	2004 Apr	
5. Habit-breaking appliances.	NTR-NR	2001 Oct	101

Brief notes

1. Thumbsucking habit?	NTR-NR	2002 Apr	97

10. Epidemiology of Malocclusion

Long essays

Short notes

Brief notes

11. Orthodontic Diagnosis

Long essays

1. Discuss the various diagnostic aids used in orthodontic.	NTR-NR	1997 Oct	115
2. Explain the various diagnostic aids used in case analysis.	NTR-OR	1997 May	116
3. Discuss in brief the various diagnostic aids used in orthodontic case analysis.	NTR-NR	1992 Nov	116
4. Discuss supplementary diagnostic aids used in orthodontics.	NTR-NR	2002 Apr	116

Short notes

1. Diagnostic aids.	NTR-NR	2006 Apr	115
2. Study models.	NTR-NR	1998 Oct	130
	NTR-NR	2001 Apr	
	NTR-NR	2004 Oct	134
3. Occlusal X-ray.	NTR-NR	2002 Oct	135
4. Occlusal radiograph.	NTR-OR	2000 Apr	
5. Ortho pantamogram.	NTR-NR	1999 Apr	
6. I-O X-rays in orthodontics.	NTR-NR	2005 Apr	134

Brief notes

1. Study models.	NTR-NR	2004 Oct	130
2. Occlusal X-ray.	NTR-NR	2002 Oct	135
3. Panoramic radiographs.	NTR-NR	2006 Apr	136

12. Cephalometrics

Long essays

Short notes

1. S-N plane.	NTR-NR	2006 Oct	154
2. ANB angle.	NTR-NR	1999 Apr	
	NTR-NR	2001 Oct	

3. FMA angle.	NTR-NR	2000 Apr	154
	NTR-NR	2001 Oct	
4. SNA angle.	NTR-NR	1991 Mar	154
	NTR-OR	1992 Nov	
	NTR-OR	1999 Oct	
5. Angle SNA.	NTR-NR	2005 Oct	154
6. Y-axis.	NTR-NR	1997 Apr	151
	NTR-NR	2003 Apr	
7. Y-axis angle.	NTR-NR	2004 Oct	
8. Cephalo-stat.	NTR-NR	2000 Apr	151
9. Tweeds triangle.	NTR-NR	2003 Apr	
	NTR-NR	2005 Apr	158
10. Cephalometrics in orthodontia.	NTR-NR	1993 May	
	NTR-OR	1995 Oct	142

Brief notes

1. EH angle.	NTR-NR	2004 Apr	
2. SNA angle.	NTR-NR	2002 Oct	154
3. ANB angle.	NTR-NR	2003 Apr	154
4. SNB angle.	NTR-NR	2004 Oct	154
5. Angle SNB.	NTR-NR	2005 Oct	154
6. Y-axis angle.	NTR-NR	2005 Apr	151
7. Registration point.	NTR-NR	2004 Apr	148
8. Inter-incisal angle.	NTR-NR	2005 Apr	151

13. Skeletal Maturity Indicators

Long essays

Short notes

1. Carpel index.	NTR-OR	1999 Oct	161
2. Hand wrist X-ray.	NTR-OR	1994 Nov	162
	NTR-NR	2001 Apr	
	NTR-NR	2003 Apr	
3. Handwrist radiography.	NTR-NR	1997 Apr	162
	NTR-OR	2001 Apr	

Brief notes

1. Carpel index.	NTR-NR	2006 Apr	161

14. Model Analysis

Long essays

Short notes

Question	University	Year	Page
1. Pont's analysis?	NTR-OR	1993 Oct	177
	NTR-NR	2005 Apr	
2. Model analysis?	NTR-NR	1990 Jul	151
	NTR-OR	1995 Oct	
	NTR-OR	1998 Apr	
	NTR-NR	2003 Apr	
3. Carey's analysis?	NTR-NR	2006 Apr	175
4. Nance cares's analysis?	NTR-NR	2002 Apr	175
5. Arch perimeter analysis?	NTR-NR	1999 Oct	175
6. Model analysis for mined dentition?	NTR-OR	1997 Apr	151
	NTR-OR	1998 Oct	

Brief notes

Question	University	Year	Page
1. Pont's model analysis?	NTR-NR	2005 Oct	177
2. Pont's analysis (post's)?	NTR-NR	2000 Apr	177
3. Carey's model analysis?	NTR-NR	2004 Oct	175

15. Biology of Tooth Movement

Long essays

Question	University	Year	Page
1. Discuss the tissue changes with orthodontic tooth movement?	NTR-OR	1990 Feb	183
2. Describe the tissue changes consequent to orthodontic forces?	NTR-OR	1993 Oct	183
3. Discuss the various tissue changes taking place during orthodontic tooth movement?	NTR-NR	2005 Apr	183

Short notes

Question	University	Year	Page
1. Ideal orthodontic force.	NTR-NR	2001 Oct	185
2. Theories of tooth movement.	NTR-OR	1998 Apr	188
3. Under mining resorption.	NTR-NR	1992 Nov	192
	NTR-OR	1995 Oct	
	NTR-OR	1997 Oct	
	NTR-OR	1998 Oct	
	NTR-NR	2006 Oct	
4. Undermining bone resorption.	NTR-NR	1994 Nov	192
	NTR-OR	1997 Oct	
	NTR-NR	2001 Oct	
5. Wolf's law of transformation of bone?	NTR-OR	1992 Nov	

Brief notes

Question	University	Year	Page
1. Wolf's law?	NTR-NR	2005 Apr	
2. Frontal resorption?	NTR-NR	2002 Apr	183

Bhalaji

3. Undermining resorption?	NTR-NR	2004 Apr	192
4. Optimum orthodontic force.	NTR-NR	2006 Apr	185
5. Tissue changes on pressure side?	NTR-NR	2005 Oct	182

16. The Mechanics of Tooth Movement

Long essays

Short notes

1. Intrusion	NTR-NR	2000 Apr	199
	NTR-NR	2001 Apr	

Brief notes

1. Intrusion	NTR-NR	2001 Apr	199

17. Anchorage

Long essays

1. Define anchorage. Explain in detail different types of anchorage with an example?	NTR-OR	1994 Nov	203, 205
2. Classify anchorage. Classify orthodontic anchorage and explain with examples?	NTR-NR	2006 Apr	205
3. Define anchorage. Discuss classification of anchorage. Explain intermaxillary anchorage.	NTR-NR	2004 Oct	203, 205

Short notes

1. Anchorage.	NTR-OR	1999 Oct	203
2. Extra oral anchorage.	NTR-NR	1993 May	206
	NTR-OR	1997 Apr	
3. Reciprocal anchorage.	NTR-NR	2001 Apr	205
	NTR-NR	2006 Oct	
4. Intermaxillary anchorage.	NTR-NR	1992 Nov	207
5. Anchorage in orthodontics.	NTR-NR	1998 Oct	203

Brief notes

18. Age Factors in Orthodontics

Long essays

Short notes

Brief notes

Bhalaji

19. Preventive Orthodontics

Long essays

Question	University	Year	Page
1. Define preventive orthodontics. Discuss the various treatment plan given under the preventive orthodontics	NTR-NR	1999 Oct	215

Short notes

Question	University	Year	Page
1. Preventive orthodontics.	NTR-NR	1994 Nov	215
	NTR-OR	1998 Apr	
	NTR-NR	2006 Oct	
2. Discuss preventive orthodontic procedures.	NTR-OR	1991 Mar	216
3. Space maintainer.	NTR-NR	2002 Oct	219
	NTR-NR	2004 May	
	NTR-NR	2005 Oct	
4. Fixed space maintainer.	NTR-NR	1997 Apr	272
5. Distal shoe space maintainer.	NTR-OR	1998 Oct	224
6. Methods of space gaining in dental arch.	NTR-NR	2006 Apr	

Brief notes

20. Interceptive Orthodontics

Long essays

Question	University	Year	Page
1. Define interceptive orthodontics. Describe in detail about social interactions.	NTR-NR	1998 Oct	227

Short notes

Question	University	Year	Page
1. Serial extractions.	NTR-OR	1992 Nov	228
	NTR-OR	1993 May	
	NTR-NR	2004 Apr	236
2. Muscle exercises.	NTR-OR	1997 Oct	

Brief notes

21. Methods of Space Gaining

Long essays

Short notes

Brief notes

22. Arch Expansion

Long essays

Short notes

1. Rapid palatal expansion.	NTR-NR	1998 Oct	232
2. Slow expansion appliance.	NTR-NR	1999 Apr	238
3. Rapid Maxillary expansion.	NTR-NR	2005 Apr	232
4. Dental Vs skeletal expansion.	NTR-OR	1991 Aug	233

Brief notes

1. RME?	NTR-NR	2006 Oct	247
2. Coffin spring.	NTR-NR	2005 Apr	256
3. Expansion appliance.	NTR-NR	2004 Oct	254
4. Expansion screws.	NTR-NR	2006 Oct	254
5. Rapid palatal expansion.	NTR-NR	2002 Apr	247

23. Extractions

Long essays

1. Describe in detail about extractions in orthodontics.	NTR-NR	1998 Oct	259
2. Describe about extractions in orthodontics, with reasons.	NTR-OR	1997 Oct	259
3. What are the reasons for extractions in orthodontics? Discuss the choice of teeth for extractions.	NTR-NR	1997 Apr	259
4. Describe in detail about extractives in orthodontics. Give your choice of teeth in extractions with reasons.	NTR-OR	2001 Apr	260
5. What are the reasons for extractions in orthodontics? Discuss the choice of teeth for extractions?	NTR-OR	1993 Oct	260

Short notes

1. Extraction in orthodontics.	NTR-NR	1999 Oct	261
2. Therapeutic extraction.	NTR-OR	1997 May	260
	NTR-NR	2005 Oct	
3. Therapeutic extraction in orthodontics.	NTR-NR	2004 Oct	261

Brief notes

24. Orthodontic Appliances—General Principles

Long essays

Short notes

1. Ideal requisites of orthodontic appliance.	NTR-NR	2004 Oct	274

Brief notes

25. Removable Orthodontic Appliances

Long essays

Short notes

1. Z spring.	NTR-OR	1990 Jul	291
2. Crozat clasp.	NTR-NR	2006 Oct	
3. Adams clasp.	NTR-NR	1995 Oct	280
	NTR-OR	1999 Oct	
4. Labial low.	NTR-OR	2001 Apr	280
5. Canine retractors.	NTR-NR	2000 Apr	286
	NTR-NR	2006 Oct	
6. Robert's retractor.	NTR-NR	1997 Oct	
7. Orthodontic springs.	NTR-NR	1998 Apr	
a. Removable appliance.	NTR-NR	1998 Apr	
b. Springs to bring about mesiodistal.	NTR-NR	1997 Apr	
c. Self-supporting springs.	NTR-NR	2004 Oct	
d. Bite plane appliances.	NTR-NR	2005 Apr	

Brief notes

1. Labial bows.	NTR-NR	2004 Apr	280
2. Coffin spring.	NTR-NR	2005 Apr	286
3. Adam's clasp.	NTR-NR	2002 Apr	280
	NTR-NR	2005 Oct	
4. High labial bow.	NTR-NR	2006 Oct	286
5. Canine retractors.	NTR-NR	2005 Oct	292
6. Orthodontic clasp.	NTR-NR	2006 Oct	
7. Bite plane appliance.	NTR-NR	2004 Oct	299
8. Components of removable appliances.	NTR-NR	2006 Apr	278
9. Advantages of removable orthodontic appliances.	NTR-NR	2005 Oct	287
10. Disadvantages of removable orthodontic appliances.	NTR-NR	2006 Apr	287

26. Fixed Orthodontic Appliances

Long essays

Short notes

1. Elastics.	NTR-NR	1999 Oct	315
2. Arch wire.	NTR-OR	1999 Oct	314
3. 18-8 stainless steel.	NTR-NR	2001 Apr	314
4. Stainless steel in orthodontics.	NTR-OR	1997 May	314
5. Fixed appliance.	NTR-NR	1997 May	301
	NTR-OR	1997 Oct	
	NTR-OR	1998 Oct	98

			Bhalaji
6. Parts of fixed appliance.	NTR-OR	2001 Apr	303
7. Components of fixed appliance.	NTR-OR	2000 Apr	309
	NTR-NR	2005 Apr	
8. Fixed appliances versus removable appliances.	NTR-OR	1997 Apr	

Brief notes

1. Elastics.	NTR-NR	2002 Apr	315
2. Parts of fixed appliance.	NTR-NR	2002 Oct	309
3. 18-8 stainless steel.	NTR-NR	2003 Apr	314
4. Advantages of fixed appliances.	NTR-NR	2004 Apr	

27. Myofunctional Appliances

Long essays

1. Explain the steps in the fortification of oral screen and give its disadvantages?	NTR-NR	2006 Oct	329
2. What are the functional appliances? Give examples. Discuss any one appliance in detail?	NTR-NR	2003 Apr	329
3. What are myofunctional appliances. Describe in detail about preparation and uses of oral screen	NTR-NR	1998 Apr	329
4. What are myofunctional appliances? Classify them. Explain activator?	NTR-NR	2004 Apr	329
5. State principles of Andersen appliance. Discuss in detail indications, contraindications, uses and construction.	NTR-OR	2000 Apr	329
6. What are functional appliances? Give examples. Describe the trimming and mechanism of action of Anderson's appliance.	NTR-OR	1997 Apr	329

Short notes

1. Oral screen?	NTR-NR	1993 Oct	335
	NTR-OR	1997 Oct	
	NTR-OR	2000 Apr	
	NTR-NR	2001 Apr	
	NTR-NR	2006 Apr	
2. Lip bumper?	NTR-NR	2003 Apr	207
3. FR II appliances?	NTR-NR	2005 Oct	350
4. Frankel's appliance?	NTR-NR	1997 Oct	350
5. Functional regulators?	NTR-NR	1997 May	350
	NTR-OR	1998 Oct	
	NTR-OR	1999 Oct	

Brief notes

1. Bionator.	NTR-NR	2006 Apr	355
2. Oral screen.	NTR-NR	2003 Apr	355
	NTR-NR	2004 Oct	
3. Classification of functional appliance.	NTR-NR	2002 Oct	355

28. Orthopedic Appliances

Long essays

Short notes

1. Head gear?	NTR-NR	2003 Apr	361

Brief notes

1. Chin cap	NTR-NR	2006 Apr	375

29. Treatment Planning

Long essays

Short notes

Brief notes

30. Management of Common Malocclusions

Long essays

1. Describe the causes of midline diastema and explain how will you correct the same?	NTR-NR	1992 Nov	385
2. Describe the causes of median diastema and the measures to correct it.	NTR-NR	1993 May	385

Short notes

1. Midline diastema.	NTR-NR	1997 Apr	385
	NTR-OR	1999 Apr	
	NTR-OR	2001 Apr	
	NTR-NR	2003 Apr	
2. Maxillary Midline diastema?	NTR-NR	2006 Apr	392
3. Midline diastema diagnosis and its causes.	NTR-NR	1993 Oct	385
4. Lower anterior crowding.	NTR-NR	2000 Apr	392

Brief notes

1. Rotation.	NTR-NR	2005 Oct	394
2. Midline diastema.	NTR-NR	2002 Apr	385

Bhalaji

31. Management of Class-II Malocclusion

Long essays

1. Discuss the treatment plan for angles class II malocclusion patients in mixed dentition period	NTR-OR	1999 Apr	
2. Discuss clinical picture of Angle's class II Div 1 malocclusion and its clinical management.	NTR-NR	2004 Apr	
3. Discuss your treatment of appliance for a patient aged 8 years, presenting class II div 1 malocclusion with positive VTO	NTR-NR	1995 Oct	
4. Describe the typical clinical features of Angle's class II, div 1 malocclusion and discuss your line of treatment for 12 years old girl with Class II, Div 1?	NTR-OR	1991 Mar	

Short notes

1. Clinical features of class II div 2.	NTR-NR	2001 Apr	405
2. Clinical features of class II div 1 malocclusion.	NTR-NR	2002 Apr	397

Brief notes

32. Management of Class-III Malocclusion

Long essays

1. Discuss the clinical picture of skeletal angle's class III malocclusion and its clinical management?	NTR-NR	2005 Oct	409

Short notes

Brief notes

33. Management of Open Bite

Long essays

Short notes

1. Open bite.	NTR-NR	1991 Mar	415
	NTR-OR	1993 May	
	NTR-NR	2005 Oct	
2. Anterior open bite.	NTR-NR	1997 Oct	415
	NTR-OR	1998 Oct	
	NTR-OR	1998 Oct	
	NTR-NR	2001 Oct	

Bhalaji

Brief notes

1. Open bite.	NTR-NR	2002 Apr	415

34. Management of Crossbite

Long essays

Short notes

1. Anterior crossbite.	NTR-NR	1999 Apr	428
	NTR-OR	1995 Oct	
2. Citoles appliance.	NTR-NR	1993 Oct	428
	NTR-OR	2001 Oct	
3. Crossbite.	NTR-NR	1997 May	428
	NTR-OR	2001 Oct	
	NTR-NR	2004 Apr	
4. Springs to bring about mesiodistal.	NTR-OR	1997 Apr	

Brief notes

1. Inclined plane?	NTR-NR	2006 Apr	
	NTR-NR	2006 Oct	
2. Posterior crossbite?	NTR-NR	2003 Apr	428

35. Management of Deep Bite

Long essays

Short notes

1. Deep bite?	NTR-NR	1999 Apr	433
	NTR-NR	2002 Oct	
2. Deep over bite?	NTR-OR	1993 Oct	433
3. Anterior deep bite?	NTR-NR	1992 Nov	437

Brief notes

36. Cleft Lip and Palate

Long essays

Short notes

1. Cleft lip and palate?	NTR-NR	2001 Apr	440
2. Management of left lip and palate?	NTR-NR	1998 Apr	444

Brief notes

1. Cleft lip	NTR-NR	2005 Apr	440

Bhalaji

37. Surgical Orthodontics

Long essays

Short notes

1. Precision?	NTR-NR	2003 Apr	454
2. Surgical orthodontics?	NTR-OR	1997 May	450
	NTR-NR	2006 Oct	
3. Supracrystal fibrotomy?	NTR-NR	2002 Apr	

Brief notes

1. Precision?	NTR-NR	2004 Oct	454

38. Retention and Relapse

Long essays

1. Discuss retention and release in orthodontics.	NTR-NR	2001 Oct	466

Short notes

1. Relapse.	NTR-NR	2001 Apr	
2. Hawley's retainer.	NTR-NR	1997 Apr	466
	NTR-OR	1998 Apr	
3. Permanent retention.	NTR-OR	2000 Apr	
4. Retention appliance.	NTR-OR	1992 Nov	
	NTR-OR	1993 May	
	NTR-OR	1995 Oct	
	NTR-NR	2006 Apr	
5. Retention and relapse.	NTR-NR	1994 Nov	
	NTR-OR	1998 Oct	
	NTR-OR	2000 Apr	
6. Retention and retainers.	NTR-NR	1998 Apr	
7. Upper Hawley's appliance.	NTR-OR	1994 Nov	

Brief notes

1. Fixed retainer.	NTR-NR	2003 Apr	468
2. Retention appliance.	NTR-NR	2002 Apr	468

39. Lab Procedures

Long essays

Short notes

1. Soldering.	NTR-NR	1993 Oct	473
	NTR-OR	1995 Oct	

2. Spot welder.	NTR-NR	1999 Oct	476
3. Study models.	NTR-NR	1998 Oct	478
	NTR-NR	2006 Oct	
4. Soldering and welding.	NTR-NR	1992 Nov	473
	NTR-OR	1993 May	
	NTR-OR	2001 Apr	
5. Welding in orthodontics.	NTR-OR	1993 Oct	476
6. Orthodontic study models.	NTR-NR	2005 Oct	478

Brief notes

1. Study models.	NTR-NR	2004 Oct	478
2. Solder and flux.	NTR-NR	2003 Apr	473
3. Dental spot welder.	NTR-NR	2001 Apr	476
4. Soldering and welding.	NTR-NR	2005 Apr	473

40. Genetics in Orthodontics

Long essays

Short notes

1. Genetics in orthodontics?	NTR-OR	1998 Oct	485
2. Role of hereditary in malocclusion?	NTR-OR	1994 Nov	488

Brief notes

41. Computers in Orthodontics

Long essays

Short notes

Brief notes

42. Adult Orthodontics

Long essays

Short notes

1. Age factors in orthodontics?	NTR-OR	2001 Oct	211

Brief notes

43. Materials Used in Orthodontics

Long essays

Short notes

Brief notes

44. Orthodontic Instruments

Long essays

Short notes

Brief notes

45. Sterilization in Orthodontics

Long essays

Short notes

Brief notes

46. Computers in Orthodontics

Long essays

Short notes

Brief notes

47. Lingual Orthodontics

Long essays

Short notes

Brief notes

48. Cosmetic Contouring in Orthodontics

Long essays

Short notes

Brief notes

49. Detrimental Effects of Orthodontic Treatment

Long essays

Short notes

Brief notes

50. Miscellaneous

Long essays

Short notes

1.	Intrusion.	NTR-OR	2000 Apr
2.	Teratogens.	NTR-OR	1999 Apr
3.	Bolton plane.	NTR-NR	2005 Apr
4.	Direct bouling.	NTR-OR	2001 Apr
5.	Capsular matrix.	NTR-OR	1994 Nov
6.	Mandibular plane.	NTR-NR	2004 Apr
7.	Sheldon body type.	NTR-NR	2001 Apr
8.	Gnatho-static models.	NTR-NR	2004 Apr
9.	Mandibular retrognathism.	NTR-NR	2004 Oct
10.	Postnatal causes for malocclusion.	NTR-NR	2002 Apr
11.	Oral hygiene measures during orthodontic treatment.	NTR-NR	1993 May

Brief notes

1.	Imbrications.	NTR-NR	2004 Apr
2.	Acromegalae.	NTR-NR	2005 Apr
3.	Interincisal angle.	NTR-NR	2005 Apr
4.	Borderline case.	NTR-NR	2001 Apr
5.	Occlusal plane.	NTR-NR	2003 Oct
6.	Mandibular plane.	NTR-NR	2005 Oct
7.	Registration point.	NTR-NR	2004 Apr
8.	Skeletal malocclusion.	NTR-NR	2001 Apr
9.	Irreversible hydrocolloids.	NTR-NR	2003 Apr

COMPLETE DENTURES

SYLLABUS

Biomechanics of the Edentulous State

- Mechanism of tooth support
- Mechanism of complete denture support
- Masticatory load and mucosal support
- Residual ridge and psychological effect on retention
- Functional and parafunctional considerations
- Functions: mastication and swallowing
- Mandibular movements
- Parafunctions and occlusion
- Distribution of stresses to the denture supporting tissues changes in morphological face height and the tempromandibular joint
- Individual behavioral or adaptive response—cosmetic changes, dietary changes, adaptive and psychological changes, adaptive potential of the patient

The Aging Edentulous Patient

- Soft tissue changes and soft tissue hyperplasia
- Denture sore mouth and denture stomatitis, treatment of denture stomatitis

Effects of Aging

- Oral changes and mucosa and skin
- Residual bone and the maxillomandibular relation
- Disuse atrophy and changes in the size of the basal seat
- Tongue and taste and dietary problems
- Salivary flow and nutritional impairment
- Degenerative changes and Psychological changes

Preparing the Patient for Complete Denture Prosthesis

- Diagnosis and treatment planning for patient with some teeth remaining
- Diagnostic procedures
- History and records
- Immediate complaints
- Systemic evaluation—CVS, respiratory, renal, endocrines, CNS and other systemic conditions
- Temporomandibular joint disorders
- Intraoral examination diagnostic cast Interarch space problems radiographs and other investigations

Treatment Plan

- Deciding whether to extract the remaining teeth
- Pre-extraction record
- The patient recently made edentulous and desires and expectations
- The patient edentulous for a long time
- Mental attitudes and classification
- The house classification and application of the house classifications

Diagnosis of Patient with No Teeth Remaining

- Examination charts and records
- General observations affecting diagnosis
- Radiographic and intraoral examination and advantages of a radiographic examination
- Intraoral examination

Communicating with the Patient

- Nutrition counseling, calcium and bone health, vitamin supplementation
- Nutrition care of the denture patient
- Nutritional needs and status of the elderly
- Impact of wearing dentures on dietary intake

Identification and Management of the Patient with Problems

- Basic rules to follow to avoid problems
- Conduction of the comprehensive examination
- Correctional procedures prior to making prosthesis
- Patient behavior characteristics observed during the examination appointment that may indicate future management problems
- Disrupting regular office routine
- Overreacting to normal examination procedures
- Downgrading or criticizing treatment provided by a previous dentist
- Refusing to divulge the name of a previous dentist or dentists
- Dissatisfaction with existing prosthesis that does not coincid with you evaluation of the prosthesis
- Numerous sets of prostheses made in a short time (for example, three in two years)

Improving the Patient's Denture Foundation and Ridge Relations

Nonsurgical Methods

- Rest for the prosthesis supporting tissues
- Occlusal and vertical dimension correcting of old prostheses
- Good nutrition and conditioning of the patient's musculature

Surgical Methods

- Correcting conditions that preclude optimal prosthetic function
- Hyperplastic ridge, epulis fissuratum, and papillomatosis
- Frenular attachments and pendulous maxillary tuberosities
- Bony prominences, undercuts, spiny ridges, and nonparallel bony ridges
- Discrepancies in jaw size
- Pressure on the mental foramen
- Enlargement of denture-bearing areas
- Vestibuloplasty
- Ridge augmentation
- Replacing tooth roots by osseointegrated dental implants
- Management of remaining teeth and pulp for over dentures

Biologic Considerations for Maxillary Impressions

- Macroscopic anatomy of supporting structures
- Support for the maxillary denture
- Residual ridge
- Stress-bearing areas
- Incisive papilla
- Posterior palatal area
- Bone of the basal seat

Macroscopic Anatomy of Limiting Structures

- Labial frenum
- Orbicularis oris
- Buccal frenum
- Buccal vestibule
- Pterygomaxillary notch
- Palatine fovea region
- Vibrating line of the palate

Microscopic Anatomy

- Histologic nature of soft tissue and bone
- Microscopic anatomy of supporting tissues
- Microscopic anatomy of limiting structures

Biologic Considerations for Mandibular Impressions

Macroscopic Anatomy of the Supporting Structures

- Crest of the residual ridge
- Buccal flange area and the buccal shelf
- Flat mandibular ridges
- Bone of the basal seat
- Stages of change in the mandible
- Mylohyoid ridge
- Throat form and tongue positions
- Mental foramen area resorption
- Insufficient space between the mandible and the tuberosity
- Low mandibular ridges
- Direction of ridge resorption
- Torus mandibularis

Macroscopic Anatomy of Limiting Structures

- Buccal and labial borders
- Buccal vestibule
- External oblique ridge and the buccal flange
- Masseter muscle region

- Distal extension of the mandibular impression
- Retromolar region and pad
- Lingual borders
- Influence and action of the floor of the mouth
- Mylohyoid muscle and mylohyoid ridge
- Sublingual gland region
- Direction of the lingual flange
- Alvcololingual sulcus
- Lingual frenum and lingual notch Lingual flange

Microscopic Anatomy

- Supporting tissues
- Crest of the residual ridge
- Buccal shelf

Impressions for the Edentulous Patient

- Primary impression—Patients position, operators position, stock trays, materials and step by step procedure for making primary impression
- Impression trays—Special trays and design for final impression
- Final impression materials

Impression Techniques

- First technique—Border molded special tray
- Second technique—One step border molded tray
- Third technique—Custom tray design based on the previously worn prosthesis

Mandibular Impression Procedures

- Classification of mandibular impressions
- Aims and objectives, and theories of impression making
- Selective pressure impressions
- Pressure less impressions
- Construction procedures
- First technique—Selective pressure mandibular impression border-molded special tray
- Second technique—Selective pressure mandibular impression-one step border-molded tray
- Third technique—Selective pressure Mandibular impression custom tray design based on the previously worn prosthesis

Biologic Considerations in Jaw Relations and Jaw Movements

- Anatomic factors temporomandibular articulation
- Classification of jaw relations
- Orientation relations and face bow
- Vertical relations
- Horizontal relations
- Movements of the mandible

Biologic Consideration in Vertical Jaw Relations

- Anatomy and physiology of vertical jaw relations
- Establishment of the vertical maxillomandibular relations for complete denture prosthesis
- Methods of determining the vertical dimension
- Mechanical methods
- Physiologic methods
- Tests of vertical jaw relations with the occlusion rims

Biologic Considerations in Horizontal Jaw Relations

- Muscle involvement in centric relations
- Harmony between centric relation and centric occlusion
- Orienting centric relation to hinge axis
- Orienting centric relation and vertical relations
- Significance of centric relation
- Recording centric relation
- Extraoral tracing and devices
- Intraoral tracing devices
- Interocclusal centric relation records

Recording and Transferring Bases and Occlusion Rims

- Trial denture base, or recording base
- Occlusion rims
- Guide for esthetics—Central line, lip line, canine line, smile line
- Level of the occlusal plane
- Preliminary centric relations records

Relating the Patient to the Articulator

- Articulators and selection of articulator for complete dentures
- Hanau articulator
- Whip mix articulator
- Dentatus articulator

Selecting Artificial Teeth for the Edentulous Patient

Anterior tooth selection

- Pre-extraction guides
- Size of the anterior teeth
- Form of the anterior teeth
- The dentogenic concept in selecting artificial teeth

Posterior Tooth Selection

- Buccolingual width of posterior teeth
- Mesiodistal length of posterior teeth
- Vertical length of the buccal surfaces of posterior teeth
- Types of posterior teeth according to materials
- Types of posterior teeth according to cusp inclines

Preliminary Arrangement of Artificial Teeth

Guides for Preliminarily Arranging Anterior Teeth

- Relationship to incisive papilla
- Relationship to the reflection
- Factors governing the anteroposterior position of the dental arch

Setting Maxillary Anterior Teeth in Wax for Try in

Importance of proper anteroposterior positioning of the anterior teeth

Setting Mandibular Anterior Teeth in the Wax for Try in

Horizontal overlap

Preliminary Arrangement of Posterior Teeth

- Orientation of occlusal plane
- Tentative buccolingual position of the posterior teeth
- Tentative arch form of the posterior teeth

Setting posterior teeth for try in

- Guidelines for centric occlusion
- Esthetics and leverage

Completion of the Try in: Eccentric Jaw Relation Records Articulators and Cast Adjustment, Establishing the Posterior Palatal Seal

- Protrusive and lateral relations
- Controlling factors of movement
- Eccentric relation records
- Establishing the posterior palatal seal

Appearance and Functional Harmony of Denture Bases

- Materials used for denture bases
- Formation and preparation of the mold packing the mold
- Preserving the orientation relations
- Construction of remounting casts
- Completing the rehabilitation of the patient
- Dentists evaluations
- Patients evaluations friends evaluations
- Treatment of the time of the denture insertion
- Elimination of basal surface errors
- Errors in occlusion
- Interocclusal records for remounting dentures
- Interocclusal record of centric relation
- Remounting the mandibular denture verifying centric relation
- Phonetics—Production of voice and articulation of sounds

- Position of teeth and phonetics
- Neutral, zone, relief
- Processing errors—Reasons and care
- Selective grinding
- Remount and correction of occlusal discrepancies
- Prosthesis—Examination insertion

Patient's Instructions after Care and Recall and Management of Patient Complaints

- Protrusive interocclusal record
- Alternative use of plaster interocclusal records advantages of balanced
- Occlusion in complete dentures special instructions to the patient
- Individuality of patients
- Appearance with new dentures
- Mastication with new dentures
- Speaking with new dentures
- Oral hygiene with dentures
- Maintaining the comfort and health of the oral cavity in a rehabilitated edentulous patient
- Adjustments relaxed to the occlusion
- Adjustments relaxed to the denture bases
- Subsequent oral examinations and treatments

Special Complete Dentures

Tooth-supported Complete Dentures

- Indications and contraindication for over dentures
- Selection of abutment teeth
- Clinical procedures

Immediate Denture Treatment

- Indication and contraindications for immediate dentures
- Treatment planning
- Clinical procedures
- Subsequent service for immediate dentures

Single Complete Dentures Opposing Natural Teeth

- Maxillary and mandibular single dentures
- Clinical and laboratory procedures
- Subsequent problems with single dentures against natural teeth

Relining or Rebasing of Complete Dentures

- Diagnosis and treatment rationale
- Clinical procedures
- Static impression technique closed and open mouth relines/rebases
- Functional impression technique
- Chair side technique

Repair of Complete Dentures and Duplication of Casts

- Maxillary and mandibular fracture repair
- Repairs using cold-curing resin
- Duplication of casts
- Reversible and Irreversible hydrocolloid technique

Osteointegrated Supported Prosthesis (Dental Implants) for the Edentulous Patients

- Maladaptive denture behavior
- Use of dental implants
- Patient considerations
- Tissue integration in the edentulous patient

Management of Japer-Plastic Ridges

- Atrophied flat mandibular ridges in complete denture prosthesis therapy.

Geriatric Dentistry

- Management of aged, senior citizens, physically, mentally handicapped patients.

Miscellaneous

- Broken prosthesis
- Swallowing prosthesis
- General management of elderly and immunocompromised patients.

SCHEME OF EXAMINATION

Theory

Theory – 70 Marks
Viva Voce – 10 Marks
Internal Assessment (Theory) – 20 Marks

Complete Dentures (Part-A + Part-B / 35 + 35 = 70)

Subject	*Type of question*	*Marks offered*	*Total*
Part-A/Complete Dentures	Long essays	9	1 x 9 = 09
	Short notes	4	4 x 4 = 16
	Brief notes	2	5 x 2 = 10
Part-B/Complete Dentures	Long essays	9	1 x 9 = 09
	Short notes	4	4 x 4 = 16
	Brief notes	2	5 x 2 = 10

Clinicals

Clinicals – 70 Marks
Viva Voce – 10 Marks
Internal Assessment (Clinicals) – 20 Marks

REFERENCE BOOK

Complete Dentures: Textbook of Complete Dentures – By Nalla Swamy

AUTHOR ABBREVIATION

Nalla: Nalla Swamy

Edition: 1st

QUESTION BANK ABBREVIATION

Question Bank

LE — Long essays
SN — Short notes
BN — Brief notes

University

NTRUHS — Nandamuri Taraka Rama Rao University of Health Sciences
NTRUHS-NR — NTRUHS–New Regulations
NTRUHS-OR — NTRUHS–Old Regulations

CONTENTS

Contd...

Contd...

COMPLETE DENTURES

Nalla

1. The Edentulous Patient

Long essays

Short notes

1. Edentulous state	NTR-OR	1990 Feb	

Brief notes

2. Biomechanics of the Edentulous State

Long essays

Short notes

1. Ridge resorption	NTR-NR	1994 May	233

Brief notes

3. The Effects of Aging on the Edentulous State

Long essays

Short notes

Brief notes

4. Temporomandibular Disorders in Edentulous Patients

Long essays

Short notes

Brief notes

5. Nutrition Care for the Denture Wearing Patients

Long essays

Short notes

Brief notes

6. Complete Denture Prosthodontics

Long essays

Nalla

Short notes

Brief notes

7. Parts of a Complete Denture

Long essays

Short notes

Brief notes

1. Polished surface.	NTR-NR	2002 Oct	5
	NTR-NR	2004 Oct	

8. Types of Complete Dentures

Long essays

Short notes

1. Metallic denture base.	NTR-NR	2001 Apr	5

Brief notes

9. Establishing a Rapport with a Patient

Long essays

Short notes

Brief notes

10. History Taking and Examination

Long essays

Short notes

1. Mental attitude of patients.	NTR-NR	2002 Apr	14
	NTR-NR	2004 Oct	

Brief notes

11. Diagnosis and Treatment Planning

Long essays

1. Diabetic patient aged 65 years with few teeth remaining comes to your dental college hospital for dental prosthesis. Discuss the treatment planning and special steps to be taken by you for the management of the patient?	NTR-OR	1991 Mar	

			Nalla

Short notes

Brief notes

12. Mouth Preparation for Edentulous Patients

Long essays

Short notes

1. Vestibuloplasty.	NTR-NR	2003 Apr	43
2. Pre-prosthetic surgery.	NTR-NR	2001 Oct	43
	NTR-NR	2002 Oct	
3. Pre-prosthetic surgical managements in complete denture.	NTR-NR	1998 Apr	43

Brief notes

13. Anatomy of Edentulous Mouth

Long essays

Short notes

Brief notes

14. Anatomical Landmarks in Maxilla

Long essays

Short notes

1. Incisive papilla.	NTR-NR	1990 Feb	54
	NTR-OR	2001 Apr	
	NTR-NR	2002 Oct	
2. Posterior palatal seal.	NTR-OR	1994 May	51
	NTR-OR	1995 Apr	
	NTR-OR	1996 Apr	
	NTR-NR	2005 Mar	
3. Primary stressbearing areas.	NTR-NR	1998 Oct	50
4. Maxillary anatomic landmarks.	NTR-NR	2005 Mar	50

Brief notes

1. Posterior palatal fecal area.	NTR-NR	2003 Apr	51
2. House's palate classification.	NTR-NR	2005 Oct	30
3. Significance of incisive papilla.	NTR-NR	2006 Apr	54

Nalla

15. Anatomical Landmarks in Mandible

Long essays

1. Discuss the anatomical landmarks in case of a completely edentulous patient?	NTR-OR	2001 Oct	50

Short notes

1. Retromolar pad.	NTR-NR	1990 Feb	57
	NTR-OR	1994 Nov	
2. Mylohyoid ridge.	NTR-NR	1990 Feb	59
3. Buccal sheet area.	NTR-NR	2002 Apr	58
4. Significance of retro molar pad.	NTR-NR	1998 Apr	57

Brief notes

1. Neutral zone.	NTR-NR	2003 Apr	
	NTR-NR	2004 Apr	
2. Buccal shelf area.	NTR-NR	2003 Apr	58

16. Aims and Objectives of Impression Taking

Long essays

1. What are the objectives of impression making and how will you achieve them during impression making?	NTR-OR	1992 May	60
2. Define the term impression in complete denture Prosthodontics classify impression techniques and explain the objectives of impression making.	NTR-NR	1995 Oct	45

Short notes

Brief notes

17. Retention of Complete Dentures

Long essays

1. Define retention stability and support in complete denture. Write in detail about the factors influencing retention.	NTR-OR	1998 Apr	60
2. Define term retention. Describe the factors of refer in complete denture.	NTR-NR	1995 Nov	60

Short notes

1. Retention in complete dentures.	NTR-NR	1997 Apr	60
	NTR-OR	2000 Apr	
	NTR-NR	2003 Apr	

			Nalla
2. Saliva its role in complete dentures.	NTR-NR	1997 Oct	60
3. Factors affecting retention in complete dentures.	NTR-OR	2001 Oct	60

Brief notes

1. Atmospheric pressure	NTR-NR	2002 Oct	62
2. Factors affecting complete denture retention	NTR-NR	2005 Mar	60

18. Stability of Complete Dentures

Long essays

Short notes

1. Stability in complete dentures	NTR-NR	1994 May	64

Brief notes

19. Support of Complete Dentures

Long essays

Short notes

Brief notes

20. Impression Trays

Long essays

Short notes

Brief notes

21. Impression Materials

Long essays

Short notes

Brief notes

1. Final impression materials for complete denture.	NTR-NR	2004 Oct	80

22. Impression Techniques

Long essays

1. Define complete denture impression. Discuss various theories of impression making.	NTR-NR	2001 Apr	45
2. What are the objectives of impression making and how will you achieve them during impression making?	NTR-OR	1992 May	60

3. Define on impression. Discuss in detail about the most widely accepted technique of making impression in complete denture treatment.	NTR-NR	2002 Oct	45
4. Define impression for complete denture and discuss in detail the anatomic structures influencing the impression of edentulous mandible.	NTR-NR	2004 Apr	45
5. Define the term impression in complete denture Prosthodontics classify impression techniques. and explain the objectives of impression making.	NTR-NR	1995 Oct	45
6. Describe the theories of impression making in complete dentures prosthodontics. Describe the impression procedure you will follow a patient with upper anterior movable flabby tissue.	NTR-NR	1996 Apr	45

Short notes

1. Pascal's law.	NTR-OR	1997 Apr	45
2. Mucostatic impression technique.	NTR-NR	2002 Apr	45
3. Selective compression theory?	NTR-OR	1998 Apr	46
4. Selective pressure theory of impression.	NTR-OR	1995 Apr	46
5. Selective pressure impression technique.	NTR-NR	2000 Apr	46
	NTR-NR	2005 Oct	
6. Controlled pressure theory of impression making.	NTR-NR	1997 Oct	46
7. Various theories of impression making of edentulous arches?	NTR-NR	2006 Apr	45

Brief notes

23. Primary and Secondary Impressions

Long essays

Short notes

Brief notes

24. Primary and Secondary Casts

Long essays

Short notes

Brief notes

25. Special Trays and Spacer Design

Long essays

Nalla

Short notes

Brief notes

26. Border Molding Techniques

Long essays

Short notes

1. Border molding in mandible? NTR-OR 1994 Nov 89

Brief notes

27. Recording Bases and Occlusal Rims

Long essays

Short notes

1. Trial denture. NTR-NR 2003 Apr

Brief notes

28. Anatomic Factors of TMJ

Long essays

Short notes

Brief notes

29. Movements of the Mandible

Long essays

Short notes

Brief notes

30. Orientation Jaw Relations

Long essays

Short notes

1. Orientation Jaw relation. NTR-NR 1997 Apr 122

Brief notes

Nalla

31. Vertical Jaw Relations

Long essays

1. What are the types of Jaw relation? Write in detail about the definition and different methods or recording vertical jaw relation.	NTR-NR	1998 Oct	121
2. Define Jaw relations. Enumerate the various Jaw relations. Mention the significance of physiologic test position. Discuss the effects of increased diagnosis decreased vertical jaw relation.	NTR-NR	1995 Apr	121

Short notes

1. Vertical dimension.	NTR-NR	1999 Apr	130
2. Increased vertical relation.	NTR-NR	2002 Apr	130
3. Physiologic rest position.	NTR-NR	2002 Apr	135
4. Decreased vertical dimension.	NTR-NR	1995 Nov	130
5. Physiologic rest position of mandible.	NTR-NR	1995 Oct	135
6. Physiologic rest position and its significance?	NTR-NR	2006 Apr	135
7. Free way space (interocclusal distance).	NTR-NR	1994 May	135
8. Pre extraction Guides hr complete delete.	NTR-NR	2004 Apr	135

Brief notes

1. Free way space.	NTR-NR	2002 Apr	136

32. Horizontal Jaw Relations

Long essays

1. Define centric relation. Describe a method for record centric relation for complete denture construction.	NTR-NR	1994 May	141
2. Define centric relation. Write in detail any one method of recording centric relation in a complete denture patient.	NTR-NR	1999 Apr	141
3. Classify Jaw relation. Define centric relation Explain its clinical significance. What are the methods for recording centric relation Explain one in detail.	NTR-NR	2004 Oct	141
4. Define the term centric relation. Mention the significance of centric Jaw relation. Enumerate the methods of recording centric relation. Describe in detail your method of recording centric jaw relation.	NTR-OR	1997 Oct	141

Short notes

1. Gothic arch tracing.	NTR-OR NTR-OR	2001 Apr 1994 May	146

			Nalla
2. Significance of centric relation.	NTR-NR	1996 Apr	139
3. Significance of recording centric relation.	NTR-NR	2000 Apr	139
4. Methods of training the patient FO retrude mandible.	NTR-NR	2004 Apr	140

Brief notes

33. Face Bow

Long essays

Short notes

1. Face bow	NTR-NR	1992 May	123
	NTR-OR	1992 Nov	
	NTR-OR	1996 Apr	
	NTR-OR	1996 Apr	
	NTR-OR	1999 Apr	
	NTR-OR	2001 Apr	
	NTR-NR	2002 Apr	
	NTR-NR	2002 Oct	
	NTR-NR	2005 Oct	

Brief notes

34. Articulators

Long essays

1. What is an articulator? Give the classification, functions and requirements of an articulator.	NTR-NR	1997 Apr	153
2. Define articulator. Mention the different types of articulators and discuss an semi adjustable articulator.	NTR-NR	2000 Apr	153

Short notes

1. Articulators	NTR-NR	1992 Nov	153
	NTR-OR	1993 May	
	NTR-OR	1995 Oct	
	NTR-NR	2005 Oct	
	NTR-NR	2006 Apr	
2. Mean value articular.	NTR-NR	2002 Apr	159
3. Anatomical articulators.	NTR-NR	1999 Apr	
4. Requirements of an articulator.	NTR-NR	1998 Apr	153
	NTR-NR	2004 Apr	

Brief notes

1. Hinge axis.	NTR-NR	2005 Apr	535

35. Anterior Teeth Selection

Long essays

1.	Describe the methods of selecting.	NTR-NR	1992 Nov	169
2.	Anterior teeth for an edentulate patient.	NTR-OR	1993 May	169
3.	Describe the principles of selection of teeth for complete denture patient.	NTR-NR	2002 Apr	169
4.	Describe the methods of selecting anterior teeth for an edentulous patient?	NTR-OR	1993 May	174

Short notes

1.	Shade selection.	NTR-NR	2001 Oct	176
		NTR-NR	2005 Mar	
2.	Dentogenic concept.	NTR-NR	2005 Mar	174
3.	Selection of anterior teeth.	NTR-NR	1999 Apr	169
		NTR-NR	2006 Apr	

Brief notes

1.	Shade selection.	NTR-NR	2005 Mar	176
2.	Dentogenic concept.	NTR-NR	2003 Apr	174

36. Posterior Teeth Selection

Long essays

1.	Describe the principles of selection of teeth for complete denture patient.	NTR-NR	2002 Apr	169

Short notes

1.	Non-anatomic tooth?	NTR-OR	1999 Apr	9

Brief notes

1.	Cusp less teeth?	NTR-NR	2002 Oct	9
2.	Posterior tooth forms?	NTR-NR	2005 Apr	178

37. Anterior Teeth Arrangement

Long essays

Short notes

1.	Principles of arrangement of teeth in complete denture.	NTR-NR	2002 Oct	198

Brief notes

38. Posterior Teeth Arrangement

Long essays

Short notes

1. Neutral zone.	NTR-NR	2003 Apr	203
	NTR-NR	2004 Apr	
2. Non-anatomic teeth.	NTR-NR	1999 Apr	9
3. Principles of arrangement of teeth in complete denture.	NTR-NR	2002 Oct	198

Brief notes

39. Concepts of Occlusions

Long essays

Short notes

Brief notes

1. Lingualized occlusion?	NTR-NR	2006 Apr	198

40. Natural and Denture Occlusion

Long essays

Short notes

Brief notes

41. Centric Occlusion

Long essays

Short notes

Brief notes

42. Balanced Occlusion

Long essays

1. Define balanced occlusion. Explain its significance. What are the factors affecting it? Explain each in detail.	NTR-NR	2005 Mar	184
2. Define balanced occlusion. Explain the rationale of balanced occlusion. Discuss the factors controlling the balanced occlusion.	NTR-OR	2002 Apr	184

Short notes

1. Condylar guidance.	NTR-NR	2000 Apr	160
2. Balanced occlusion.	NTR-NR	1990 Feb	184
	NTR-OR	1992 Nov	
	NTR-OR	1993 May	
	NTR-OR	1994 Nov	
	NTR-OR	1995 Nov	
3. Compensating curves.	NTR-OR	1992 May	184
4. Rationale of balanced occlusion.	NTR-NR	2001 Apr	184
5. Bennet movement and Bennet angle.	NTR-NR	1992 Nov	133
	NTR-OR	1993 May	

Brief notes

1. Christensen's phenomenon.	NTR-NR	2005 Oct	166
2. Enumerate the factor affecting balanced occlusion.	NTR-NR	2006 Apr	247

43. Try-in

Long essays

Short notes

1. Try in procedure	NTR-NR	1999 Apr	206

Brief notes

44. Speech Considerations

Long essays

Short notes

Brief notes

45. Lab Procedures Prior to Denture Insertion

Long essays

Short notes

Brief notes

46. Denture Insertion

Long essays

1. Discuss in detail about insertion, instructions and after care of the complete denture.	NTR-NR	2003 Apr	219

Short notes

Brief notes

47. Patient Education and Instructions

Long essays

Short notes

1. Importance of patient education?	NTR-OR	1993 May	222
2. Instruction to patients receiving complete dentures	NTR-NR	1997 Apr	222
	NTR-OR	1998 Apr	
3. Instructions to be given to patient receiving complete denture?	NTR-OR	1995 Oct	222

Brief notes

48. Postinsertion Phase and Management

Long essays

1. Discuss in detail about insertion, instructions and after care of complete denture.	NTR-NR	2003 Apr	222
2. Discuss in detail various postinsertion problems in edentulous patients using complete dentures.	NTR-NR	2006 Apr	223
3. What are the various postinsertion problems in complete denture? Enumerate the reasons for it and their management?	NTR-NR	2005 Oct	223
4. Discuss in brief the postinsertion management in complete denture prosthodontics?	NTR-OR	1990 Feb	223

Short notes

1. Denture cleansing agents?	NTR-OR	2001 Oct	

Brief notes

49. Sequelae Caused by Wearing Complete Dentures

Long essays

Short notes

Brief notes

1. Epulis fissuratum	NTR-NR	2002 Apr	

50. Single Complete Dentures

Long essays

Nalla

Short notes

1. Single dentures.	NTR-OR	1992 Nov	250
	NTR-OR	1993 May	
2. Drawbacks of single complete denture.	NTR-NR	2002 Oct	251
3. Problems encountered in single denture construction.	NTR-OR	2000 Apr	252

Brief notes

51. Overdenture

Long essays

Short notes

1. Overdenture	NTR-NR	1992 May	259
	NTR-OR	1992 Nov	
	NTR-OR	1995 Oct	
	NTR-OR	1996 Apr	
	NTR-NR	2005 Oct	
2. Advantages of overdenture	NTR-NR	2001 Apr	260

Brief notes

1. Overdenture	NTR-NR	2004 Oct	259
2. Types of bar retained overdentures?	NTR-NR	2006 Apr	

52. Immediate Dentures

Long essays

Short notes

1. Immediate dentures.	NTR-NR	1992 May	255
	NTR-OR	1992 Nov	
2. Immediate complete denture.	NTR-NR	1994 May	255
	NTR-OR	1995 Apr	
3. Indication of immediate denture.	NTR-NR	2002 Apr	256
4. Advantages of immediate denture.	NTR-NR	2002 Apr	255
5. Advantages and disadvantages of immediate denture.	NTR-NR	2004 Oct	255
6. Immediate dentures—their advantages and disadvantages.	NTR-NR	1996 Apr	255
7. Rationale and advantages of immediate complete denture.	NTR-NR	2004 Apr	255

Brief notes

1. Advantages of immediate complete dentures?	RGUHS	2006 Apr	

Nalla

53. Implant Dentures

Long essays

Short notes

1. Implant dentures.	NTR-NR	1992 May	262
	NTR-OR	1992 Nov	
	NTR-OR	1994 May	
2. Types of implant denture.	NTR-NR	2004 Apr	262

Brief notes

54. Other Special Complete Dentures

Long essays

Short notes

1. Obturators.	NTR-NR	1992 Nov	706
	NTR-OR	1994 Nov	
	NTR-OR	1995 Apr	
	NTR-OR	1997 Oct	
	NTR-OR	2000 Apr	
	NTR-NR	2002 Apr	
	NTR-NR	2002 Oct	
	NTR-NR	2004 Oct	
2. Implant denture.	NTR-OR	1992 May	262
3. Hybrid dentures.	NTR-OR	1992 Nov	
	NTR-OR	1993 May	
4. Immediate obturator.	NTR-NR	1998 Oct	
5. Transitional denture.	NTR-NR	1994 Nov	
	NTR-OR	1995 Nov	264

Brief notes

1. Transitional denture.	NTR-NR	2002 Apr	464

55. Relining and Rebasing

Long essays

Short notes

1. Relining and rebasing.	NTR-NR	1995 Oct	239
	NTR-OR	1996 Apr	
2. Relining and rebasing of complete denture.	NTR-NR	1998 Oct	239
3. Indications diagnosis contraindications for reliving diagnosis rebasing.	NTR-NR	2005 Mar	

			Nalla

Brief notes

1. Steps in rebasing of complete dentures. NTR-NR 2004 Apr 248

56. Repair of Complete Dentures

Long essays

Short notes

Brief notes

57. Tissue Conditioners

Long essays

Short notes

1. Tissue conditioner. NTR-NR 1995 Apr 224
NTR-OR 1998 Oct
NTR-NR 2002 Apr

Brief notes

1. Tissue conditioners. NTR-NR 2000 Oct 224
NTR-NR 2004 Apr

58. Resilient Denture Liners

Long essays

Short notes

1. Resilient liners? NTR-OR 1997 Oct

Brief notes

59. Denture Adhesive Materials

Long essays

Short notes

Brief notes

60. Miscellaneous Topics

Long essays

Short notes

1. Die spacers? NTR-NR 2003 Apr
2. Pascal's law? NTR-OR 1997 Apr

	Nalla	
3. Altered cast?	NTR-NR	2002 Apr
4. Altered cast technique?	NTR-OR	1992 Oct
	NTR-OR	1997 Oct
5. Split cast technique?	NTR-OR	1990 Feb
6. Laboratory remounting?	NTR-NR	2003 Apr
7. Clinical remount procedure?	NTR-OR	1997 Apr
8. Interocclusal recording media?	NTR-NR	2003 Apr
9. Pre-extraction guides for complete denture fabrication?	NTR-NR	2004 Apr
10. Methods of training the patient to retrude the mandible?	NTR-NR	2004 Apr

Brief notes

1. Realeff effect?	NTR-NR	2004 Oct
2. Occlusal pivots?	NTR-NR	2002 Apr
3. Clinical remounting?	NTR-NR	2002 Oct
4. Define and mention the factors of dentogenics?	NTR-NR	2004 Apr

REMOVABLE PARTIAL DENTURES

SYLLABUS

1. Periodontal aspects of partial dentures.
2. Systemic methods of designing partial denture bases in relation to anatomical and histological structures of the mouth, bearing and nonbearing areas.
3. Selection and types of bars and saddle and their location, variations as per classifications in designs.
4. Effects of components of vertical forces—rotatory movement.
5. Bone resorption and reduction of vertical load distribution of the load and stress breaking principles.
6. Choice between stress breaking and rigid methods. Load distribution by mucocompression. Choice of various components.
7. Examination of the patient—oral examination, recording data, pulp tests.
8. Examination of the factors related to fixed partial denture prosthesis—position, size of the teeth, occlusion, periodontal status, perio-prosthetic considerations.

SCHEME OF EXAMINATION

Theory

Theory – 70 Marks
Viva Voce – 10 Marks
Internal Assessment (Theory) – 20 Marks

Removable Partial Dentures (Part-A + Part-B / 35 + 35 = 70)

Subject	*Type of question*	*Marks offered*	*Total*
Part-A/Removable Partial Dentures	Long essays	9	1 x 9 = 09
	Short notes	4	4 x 4 = 16
	Brief notes	2	5 x 2 = 10
Part-B/Removable Partial Dentures	Long essays	9	1 x 9 = 09
	Short notes	4	4 x 4 = 16
	Brief notes	2	5 x 2 = 10

Clinicals

Clinicals – 70 Marks
Viva Voce – 10 Marks
Internal Assessment (Clinicals) – 20 Marks

REFERENCE BOOK

Removable Partial Dentures: Textbook of Removable Partial Dentures – By Deepak Nalla Swamy

AUTHOR ABBREVIATION

Nalla: Deepak Nalla Swamy

Edition: 1st

QUESTION BANK ABBREVIATION

Question Bank

LE — Long essays
SN — Short notes
BN — Brief notes

University

NTRUHS — Nandamuri Taraka Rama Rao University of Health Sciences
NTRUHS-NR — NTRUHS–New Regulations
NTRUHS-OR — NTRUHS–Old Regulations

CONTENTS

REMOVABLE PARTIAL DENTURES

Nalla

1. Introduction to Removable Partial Dentures (RPD)

Long essays

Short notes

Brief notes

2. Parts of a Removable Partial Denture

Long essays

Short notes

Brief notes

3. Types of Removable Partial Dentures

Long essays

Short notes

1. Immediate partial denture? NTR-OR 2002 Oct 472

Brief notes

4. Partially Edentulous—Epidemiology, Physiology and Terminology

Long essays

Short notes

Brief notes

5. Clasp-retained Partial Dentures

Long essays

Short notes

Brief notes

6. Classification of Partially Edentulous Arches

Long essays

Question	University	Date	Page
1. Describe the Kennedy's classification of partially edentulous arches along with the rules governing the classification – Draw diagrams.	NTR-OR	1995 Oct	271
2. Discuss importance of diagnostic and treatment planning in removable partial denture prosthodontics. Enumerate Applegate's rule for applying the Kennedy's classification.	NTR-OR	1990 Feb	272

Short notes

Question	University	Date	Page
1. Kennedy's classification.	NTR-OR	2000 Apr	271
2. Classification of partially edentions arches.	NTR-NR	2005 Mar	270
3. Limitations of Kennedy's classification of partially edentulous spaces.	NTR-NR	2003 Apr	
4. Applegate rules for Kennedy's classification of partially edentions arches.	NTR-OR	1998 Apr	273
	NTR-NR	2005 Mar	

Brief notes

7. Biomechanics of Removable Partial Dentures

Long essays

Short notes

Brief notes

Question	University	Date	Page
1. Fulcrum line?	NTR-NR	2003 Apr	371

8. Major Connectors and Minor Connectors

Long essays

Question	University	Date	Page
1. Define major connector. Write in detail about requirements and types of mandibular major connectors?	NTR-NR	2004 Apr	327
	NTR-NR	2005 Oct	
2. Define major corrector. What are the design, requirement for major connection? Discuss in detail the mandibular major connector	NTR-OR	1995 Apr	327
3. Classify major connectors and discuss the role of major connector in removable partial dentures prosthodontics?	NTR-OR	1991 Mar	327

				Nalla

Short notes

1. Major connector	NTR-OR	1992 Nov	237
	NTR-OR	1993 May	
2. Minor connectors	NTR-OR	1997 Oct	340
	NTR-OR	1995 Apr	
	NTR-NR	2005 Apr	
3. Major connector in maxilla	NTR-OR	1994 Nov	329
	NTR-OR	1995 Nov	
4. Maxillary major connectors	NTR-NR	2005 Mar	329
	NTR-NR	2006 Apr	
5. Posterior palatal bar?	NTR-NR	2001 Oct	330
6. Lingual bar?	NTR-NR	2001 Oct	336
7. Minor connector in partial denture	NTR-OR	1994 May	340
8. U-Shaped or horse-shoe shaped major connector	NTR-NR	2004 Apr	332

Brief notes

1. Minor connectors	NTR-NR	2005 Mar	340

9. Rests and Rest seats

Long essays

Short notes

1. Occlusal rest	NTR-OR	1990 Feb	347
	NTR-OR	1992 May	
	NTR-OR	1992 Nov	
2. Rests in RPD.	NTR-NR	2005 Oct	345
3. Functions of occlusal rest	NTR-OR	1998 Apr	347
4. Occlusal rest seat preparation	NTR-OR	2002 Apr	347
5. Occlusal rest – functions diagnosis rest seat preparation	NTR-OR	1995 Apr	

Brief notes

10. Direct Retainers and Indirect Retainers

Long essays

1. Define indirect retainer. Describe the indications and reasons for the use of indirect retainer and its requirements.	NTR-OR	1998 Apr	371
2. What is direct retainer? Describe the parts of direct retainer. What are the requirements of a ideal clasp design.	NTR-OR	1997 Oct	351

3. Define a removable partial denture. How do you choose a direct retainer for a removable partial denture case?	NTR-NR	2002 Oct	351

Short notes

1. Indirect retainer	NTR-OR	1992 Nov	371
	NTR-OR	1993 May	
	NTR-OR	1994 Nov	
	NTR-OR	1997 Apr	
	NTR-OR	1995 Nov	
2. Direct retainers in RPD	NTR-OR	1998 Apr	351
3. Ring class	NTR-OR	1999 Apr	361
4. Acres clasp.	NTR-NR	2002 Apr	359
5. Combination clasp	NTR-OR	1994 Nov	362
	NTR-OR	1998 Oct	
6. Classification of clasp	NTR-OR	1998 Nov	351
7. Direct retainers (Clasp)	NTR-OR	1992 Nov	351
	NTR-OR	1996 Apr	
8. Gingivally approaching clasp	NTR-NR	2001 Apr	363
9. Factors governing clasp design?	NTR-OR	1995 Oct	354
10. Direct and indirect retention?	NTR-NR	2003 Apr	370
11. Direct retainers in removable partial dentures?	NTR-NR	2003 Apr	351

Brief notes

1. Clasp assembly?	NTR-NR	2002 Apr	352
2. Ring clasp?	NTR-NR	2003 Apr	361
3. Half and half claps?	NTR-NR	2002 Oct	362
4. Indications of embrasure clasp?	NTR-NR	2004 Apr	360

11. Stress Breakers and Precision Attachments

Long essays

Short notes

1. Stress breaker	NTR-OR	1994 Nov	393
	NTR-OR	1997 Apr	
2. Stress breaking principle?	NTR-NR	2001 Oct	393
3. Shell breakers in partial denture	NTR-OR	1994 May	393
4. Disadvantages of stress breakers	NTR-OR	1998 Oct	394

Brief notes

1. Stress breakers?	NTR-NR	2002 Oct	393

			Nalla

12. Denture Base Considerations

Long essays

Short notes

Brief notes

13. Principles of Removable Partial Denture Design

Long essays

1. Discuss various components of removable partial denture designed for Kennedy's class II situation	NTR-NR	2002 Apr	
2. Enumerate the components of removable partial denture, discuss the principles of partial denture design	NTR-OR	1992 Nov	
	NTR-OR	1993 May	
3. Discuss various components of removable partial denture and designed for Kennedy's class II situation?	NTR-NR	2002 Apr	380

Short notes

1. Problems encountered in distal extension partial denture?	NTR-NR	2002 Apr	

Brief notes

1. Fulcrum line.	NTR-NR	2003 Apr	371

14. Surveyor and Surveying Procedures

Long essays

1. Describe a dental cast surveyor. Describe the factor responsible for the path of insertion of a removable partial denture	NTR-OR	1992 Nov	307
2. Define a surveyor. Mention its parts. Explain in detail step-by-step procedure in surveying?	NTR-NR	2004 Oct	307
3. Describe a dental cast surveyor. Describe the factors responsible for the path of insertion of a removable partial denture?	NTR-OR	1992 May	307

Short notes

1. Surveyor	NTR-NR	2002 Apr	307
	NTR-OR	1990 Feb	
	NTR-NR	2003 Apr	
2. Surveying	NTR-OR	2000 Apr	307
3. Surveying tools	NTR-NR	2001 Apr	307

4. Surveying lines.	NTR-NR	2001 Oct	310
	NTR-NR	2002 Apr	
	NTR-NR	2005 Oct	
5. Dental surveyor	NTR-OR	1990 Feb	307
	NTR-OR	1995 Apr	
6. Dental cast surveyor	NTR-OR	1996 Apr	307
	NTR-OR	1995 Apr	
7. Dental model surveyor.	NTR-NR	2006 Apr	307

Brief notes

1. Tripoding?	NTR-NR	2003 Apr	316
2. Uses of dental model surveyor?	NTR-NR	2004 Apr	313

15. Treating the Partially Edentulous Patient

Long essays

Short notes

Brief notes

16. History, Examination, Diagnosis and Prognosis

Long essays

1. Discuss importance of diagnostic and treatment planning in removable partial denture prosthodontics. Enumerate Applegate's rule for applying the Kennedy's classification	NTR-OR	1990 Feb	271

Short notes

Brief notes

17. Mouth Preparation for Removable Partial Dentures

Long essays

Short notes

1. Mouth preparation in RPD.	NTR-OR	2000 Apr	300
2. Mouth preparations in removable partial dentures	NTR-OR	1997 Apr	300

Brief notes

18. Preparation of Abutment Teeth

Long essays

Short notes

Brief notes

Nalla

19. Impression Procedures for RPD

Long essays

Short notes

1. Physiological impression in RPD.	NTR-NR	2005 Apr	412
2. Impression procedure for distal extension PD.	NTR-OR	1998 Oct	410

Brief notes

20. Support for the Distal Extension Denture Base

Long essays

Short notes

Brief notes

21. Occlusal Relationship for RPD

Long essays

Short notes

Brief notes

22. Laboratory Procedures

Long essays

Short notes

Brief notes

23. Work Authorization for RPD

Long essays

Short notes

Brief notes

24. Initial Placement, Adjustments and Surveying of the RPD

Long essays

Short notes

Brief notes

25. Relining and Rebasing the RPD

Long essays

Short notes

Brief notes

26. Temporary Removable Partial Dentures

Long essays

Short notes

Brief notes

27. Removable Partial Denture Considerations in Maxillofacial Prosthesis

Long essays

Short notes

Brief notes

28. Removable Partial Over Denture

Long essays

Short notes

Brief notes

29. Glossary of Prosthodontic Terms

Long essays

Short notes

Brief notes

30. Miscellaneous

Long essays

Short notes

1.	Splints?	NTR-OR	1999 Apr
2.	Surgical splints?	NTR-OR	1998 Apr
3.	Guide planes	NTR-OR	1997 Oct
4.	Path of insertion?	NTR-OR	1995 Oct
5.	Kelly's combination syndrome?	NTR-NR	2005 Apr

Nalla

6. Key and key way attachment?	NTR-OR	1996 Apr
7. Block out procedure in cast partial denture?	NTR-NR	2002 Oct
8. Soldering and its implications and procedures?	NTR-OR	1998 Oct
9. Soldering and its applications and procedures?	NTR-OR	1997 Apr
10. Pain control in tooth preparation for retained prosthesis?	NTR-OR	1998 Oct
11. Path of insertion of removable partial dentures?	NTR-OR	1997 Apr
	NTR-OR	1999 Apr

Brief notes

1. Tensofriction?	NTR-NR	2004 Oct
2. Refractory cast?	NTR-NR	2002 Apr
3. Reciprocation in RPD?	NTR-NR	2004 Oct
4. Enameloplasty in RPD?	NTR-NR	2004 Oct

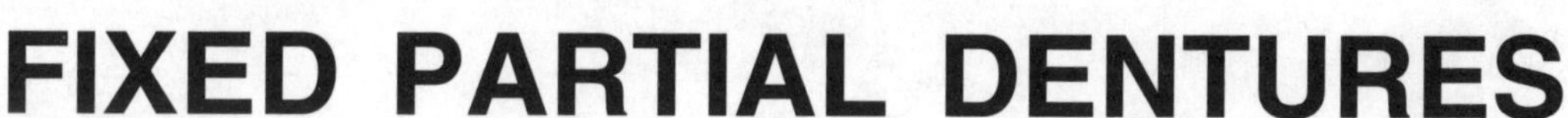

FIXED PARTIAL DENTURES

SYLLABUS

1. Planning fixed partial dentures—hygiene, therapeutic considerations, oral anatomy, normal and traumatic occlusion.
2. Histological structures of teeth and supporting tissues in relation to crowns and bridges. Passive and active eruption, gingival crevice, epithelial attachment, supporting apparatus of the teeth.
3. Principles of cavity preparation as applicable to crown and bridge prosthesis.
4. Biological interpretations of physical and mechanical principles. Types of stress, teeth as lever, stress of mastication, effects of biting forces, anterior component of force.
5. Principles of preparation of retainers. Complete and partial veneer crown, porcelain to metal restoration. Extracoronal and intracranial and radicular retainers.
6. Classification of pontics and construction.
7. Biological reactions to porcelain—root extension pontic.
8. Maintenance of fixed partial dentures. Instruction to the care and maintenance of prosthetic patient.
9. Removal and repair of crown and fixed restorations.
10. Latest trends in materials and techniques in fixed prosthodontics.

SCHEME OF EXAMINATION

Theory

Theory	–	70 Marks
Viva Voce	–	10 Marks
Internal Assessment (Theory)	–	20 Marks

Fixed Partial Dentures (Part-A + Part-B / 35 + 35 = 70)

Subject	*Type of question*	*Marks offered*	*Total*
Part-A/Fixed Partial Dentures	Long essays	9	1 x 9 = 09
	Short notes	4	4 x 4 = 16
	Brief notes	2	5 x 2 = 10
Part-B/Fixed Partial Dentures	Long essays	9	1 x 9 = 09
	Short notes	4	4 x 4 = 16
	Brief notes	2	5 x 2 = 10

Clinicals

Clinicals	–	70 Marks
Viva Voce	–	10 Marks
Internal Assessment (Clinicals)	–	20 Marks

REFERENCE BOOK

Fixed Partial Dentures: Textbook of Fixed Partial Dentures – By Deepak Nalla Swamy

AUTHOR ABBREVIATION

Nalla: Deepak Nalla Swamy

Edition: 1st

QUESTION BANK ABBREVIATION

Question Bank

LE — Long essays
SN — Short notes
BN — Brief notes

University

NTRUHS — Nandamuri Taraka Rama Rao University of Health Sciences
NTRUHS-NR — NTRUHS–New Regulations
NTRUHS-OR — NTRUHS–Old Regulations

CONTENTS

Contd...

Contd...

FIXED PARTIAL DENTURES

Nalla

1. Introduction to Fixed Partial Dentures (FPD)

Long essays

1. Describe the advantages and disadvantages of fixed partial prosthodontics? NTR-OR 1994 Nov 491

Short notes

Brief notes

2. Parts of a Fixed Partial Denture

Long essays

Short notes

Brief notes

3. Types of Fixed Partial Dentures

Long essays

Short notes

1. Maryland bridges? NTR-OR 1990 Feb 610
   NTR-OR 1997 Apr

Brief notes

4. History, Examination, Diagnosis and Prognosis

Long essays

Short notes

1. Significance of radiographs in fixed partial denture? NTR-OR 1997 Oct 492
2. Importance of radiographs in crown and bridge? NTR-OR 1994 May 492

Brief notes

5. Abutment Tooth and Periodontal Considerations

Long essays

1.	Define the term "Abutment" in fixed partial dentures. Describe the factors responsible for selection of an abutment?	NTR-NR	1996 Apr	491

Short notes

Brief notes

6. Abutment Tooth Selection and Treatment Planning

Long essays

Short notes

1.	Ante's law?	NTR-NR	2001 Oct	524
2.	Bridge abutment?	NTR-NR	1995 Oct	522
3.	Abutment selection?	NTR-NR	2004 Oct	522
4.	Selection of bridge abutment?	NTR-OR	1992 May	522
5.	Factors affecting selection of abutment tooth?	NTR-NR	2004 Apr	522

Brief notes

1.	Ante's law?	NTR-NR	2002 Oct	524
		NTR-NR	2004 Oct	
2.	Pier abutment?	NTR-NR	2005 Oct	550

7. Principles of Occlusion

Long essays

Short notes

Brief notes

1.	Types of occlusion in FPD?	NTR-NR	2005 Oct	528

8. Mouth Preparation

Long essays

1.	Discuss the mouth preparation of a patient for fixed partial denture?	NTR-OR	2001 Oct

Short notes

Brief notes

Nalla

9. Biomechanical Principles of Tooth Preparation

Long essays

1.	What are the principles in tooth preparation? Explain each in detail?	NTR-NR	2005 Apr	567
2.	Discuss the principles of tooth preparation to receive artificial crown.	NTR-NR	2001 Apr	567
3.	List the principles of tooth preparation. Describe each with examples and instructions.	NTR-NR	1997 Apr	567
4.	Describe in detail about the steps in preparation of tooth for receiving full metal crown.	NTR-NR	2006 Apr	567
5.	Describe the principles of abutment preparation for fixed partial denture.	NTR-NR	2003 Apr	567
6.	Discuss the biomechanical principles of tooth reduction in fixed partial denture prosthodontics.	NTR-OR	1990 Feb	567

Short notes

1.	Shoulder	NTR-NR	1994 May	572
2.	Finish lines?	NTR-OR	1990 Feb	571
3.	Finish lines in FPD?	NTR-NR	2004 Oct	571
4.	Finish line—location and types?	NTR-OR	1995 Oct	571
5.	Gingival finish lines?	NTR-NR	1998 Apr	571
6.	Marginal finish lines?	NTR-NR	2002 Apr	571
7.	Axioproximal grooves?	NTR-OR	1998 Apr	571
		NTR-NR	2001 Oct	
8.	Principles of tooth preparation?	NTR-NR	1998 Apr	567
9.	Types of gingival finish lines in crown preparation?	NTR-NR	1992 Nov	571

Brief notes

1.	Chamfer?	NTR-NR	2001 Oct	571
		NTR-NR	2002 Oct	
2.	Shoulder?	NTR-NR	2003 Apr	571
3.	Disadvantages of subgingival finishing lines?	NTR-NR	2006 Apr	571

10. The Complete Cast Crown Preparation

Long essays

Short notes

Brief notes

Nalla

11. The Metal Ceramic Cast Crown Preparation

Long essays

Short notes

1. Metal crown?	NTR-NR NTR-OR	1996 Apr 1999 Apr	606
2. PFM (porcelain fused to metal restoration)?	NTR-NR	2000 Apr	606

Brief notes

12. Partial Veneer Crown, Inlay and Onlay Preparations

Long essays

1. Discuss the principles of preparation of abutment teeth for partial veneer crown.	NTR-NR	1999 Apr	585

Short notes

1. Partial veneer crown	NTR-NR	1999 Apr	585
2. Proximal groves in partial veneer crown?	NTR-OR	1994 Nov	585
3. Indications, advantages and disadvantages of 3/4th partial veneer crown?	NTR-NR	2004 Apr	

Brief notes

1. Disadvantages of partial veneer crown?	NTR-NR	2005 Apr	

13. Tooth Preparation for All Ceramic Restorations

Long essays

1. Define retainer in FPD. Classify the retainers in FPD and describe the step by step preparation of posterior tooth to receive a complete veneer crown.	NTR-NR	1998 Oct	

Short notes

1. Full veneer crown.	NTR-NR	1997 Oct	575
2. Porcelain jacket crown.	NTR-NR	1995 Apr	575
3. Advantages of porcelain jacket crown.	NTR-NR	1999 Apr	601

Brief notes

1. Jacket crown?	NTR-NR	2003 Apr	575
2. Advantages of porcelain jacket crown?	NTR-NR	2002 Apr	601

14. Restoration of Endodontically Treated Tooth

Long essays

Short notes

1. Post and crown.	NTR-NR	1997 Oct	555
2. Dowel crown.	NTR-NR	1999 Apr	555

Brief notes

			Nalla

15. Implant Supported Fixed Prostheses

Long essays

Short notes

Brief notes

16. Impression Taking and Gingival Retraction Procedures

Long essays

1. Describe the technique of impression making in fixed partial denture treatment?	NTR-NR	2002 Apr	636

Short notes

1. Gingival retraction?	NTR-NR	1992 Nov	623
	NTR-OR	1995 Oct	
	NTR-OR	1995 Apr	
	NTR-OR	1996 Apr	
	NTR-OR	1998 Oct	
	NTR-OR	2001 Oct	
	NTR-NR	2002 Oct	
2. Impression materials in FPD?	NTR-NR	2004 Oct	632
3. Rubber base impression materials?	NTR-NR	2000 Apr	
4. Double impression technique in FPD?	NTR-OR	1998 Oct	
5. Impression procedures in fixed partial denture	NTR-NR	1998 Apr	622
	NTR-OR	1995 Mar	

Brief notes

1. Reversible colloid?	NTR-NR	2005 Apr	
2. Retraction cord?	NTR-NR	2004 Oct	624
3. Purpose of gingival retraction?	NTR-NR	2004 Apr	624

17. Provisional Restorations / Temporization

Long essays

Short notes

1. Temporization.	NTR-NR	1995 Oct	639
2. Provisional restoration.	NTR-NR	2002 Oct	639
	NTR-NR	2005 Oct	
3. Temporary tooth protection.	NTR-NR	1992 Nov	639
	NTR-OR	1993 May	

Brief notes

18. Working Casts and Dies

Long essays

Short notes

Brief notes

19. Wax Patterns

Long essays

Short notes

Brief notes

20. Design of a Fixed Partial Denture

Long essays

Short notes

Brief notes

21. Pontic Design

Long essays

1. Define pontic and classify.	NTR-NR	1994 May	506

Short notes

1. Pontic?	NTR-NR	2002 Apr	506
2. Pontics?	NTR-NR	1992 Nov	506
	NTR-OR	1993 May	
	NTR-OR	1995 Oct	
	NTR-NR	2004 Oct	
3. Hygienic pontic?	NTR-NR	2002 Apr	511
4. Root extension pontic?	NTR-OR	2001 Oct	511
5. Modified ridge lap pontic?	NTR-NR	2004 Apr	510
6. Disadvantages of ridge lap type pontic?	NTR-NR	2001 Apr	510

Brief notes

1. Hygienic pontic.	NTR-NR	2005 Oct	511

22. Bridges and Retainers

Long essays

1. Define fixed partial denture, mention the different types of retainers and the criteria for the selection of the retainers. Add a note on care for the prosthesis.	NTR-OR	2000 Apr	490, 503

Short notes

1. Bridge retainer?	NTR-NR	1992 Nov	503
	NTR-OR	1993 May	
2. Maryland bridges?	NTR-OR	1990 Feb	610
	NTR-OR	1997 Apr	

Brief notes

23. Connectors and Veneers for FPD

Long essays

Short notes

1. Connectors in FPD	NTR-NR	1997 Oct	515
2. Adhesive bridge?	NTR-OR	2001 Apr	
3. Connectors in fixed partial dentures?	NTR-NR	2006 Apr	515
4. Non-rigid connectors in crown and bridge?	NTR-OR	1994 May	516

Brief notes

1. Connectors in FPD.	NTR-NR	2005 Oct	515

24. Color Science and Shade Selection

Long essays

Short notes

Brief notes

25. Investing and Casting

Long essays

Short notes

Brief notes

1. Casting defects?	NTR-NR	2005 Apr
2. Suck back porosity?	NTR-NR	2006 Apr

26. Metal Ceramic Restoration Fabrication

Long essays

Short notes

1. Metal ceramic crown?	NTR-OR	1999 Apr	606
2. PFM (Porcelain fused metal restoration)?	NTR-OR	2000 Apr	606

Brief notes

Nalla

27. All-Ceramic Restoration Fabrication

Long essays

1. Describe the clinical and laboratory steps in the preparation of a porcelain jacket crown.	NTR-OR	1995 Sep	575

Short notes

1. Porcelain jacket crown?	NTR-OR	1995 Apr	575
2. Advantages of porcelain jacket crown?	NTR-NR	2002 Apr	601

Brief notes

1. Jacket crown?	NTR-NR	2002 Apr	575

28. Resin-retained Fixed Partial Dentures

Long essays

Short notes

Brief notes

29. Finishing the Cast Restoration

Long essays

Short notes

Brief notes

30. Communicating with the Dental Laboratory

Long essays

Short notes

Brief notes

31. Try-in, Staining and Glazing

Long essays

Short notes

Brief notes

32. Luting Agents and Cementation Procedures

Long essays

			Nalla

Short notes

1. Luting agents in FPD?	NTR-NR	2005 Oct	672
2. Luting cements for FPD?	NTR-NR	2004 Apr	672

Brief notes

1. Tooth colored cements for all porcelain crowns?	NTR-NR	2006 Apr	674

33. Follow-up Care

Long essays

Short notes

Brief notes

34. Dicor Crowns

Long essays

Short notes

Brief notes

35. Cerestore Crowns

Long essays

Short notes

Brief notes

36. Interocclusal Records

Long essays

Short notes

Brief notes

37. Occlusal Equilibration

Long essays

Short notes

Brief notes

38. Coronal Radicular Stabilization

Long essays

Short notes

Brief notes

39. Fixed Removable Prosthodontics

Long essays

Short notes

Brief notes

40. Miscellaneous Topics

Long essays

Short notes

1. Splints?	NTR-OR	1994 May	609
2. Ceramics?	NTR-NR	2005 Oct	
3. Porcelain teeth?	NTR-OR	1999 Apr	378
4. Veneering materials?	NTR-NR	2006 Apr	

Brief notes

1. Dicor?	NTR-NR	2002 Oct	
2. Cerestore?	NTR-NR	2003 Apr	
3. Nickel-chromium alloy?	NTR-NR	2002 Apr	641
4. Prothero's cone theory?	NTR-NR	2006 Apr	
5. Solders for dental cast units assembly?	NTR-NR	2006 Apr	
6. Enumerate tooth colored veneering material?	NTR-NR	2004 Apr	